LIVING
LONGER
STRONGER

Most Perigee Books are available at special quantity discounts for bulk purchases for sales promotions, premiums, fund-raising or educational use. Special books, or book excerpts, can also be created to fit specific needs.

For details, write: Special Markets: The Berkley Publishing Group, 375 Hudson Street, New York, New York 10014.

LIVING LONGER STRONGER

THE 6-WEEK PLAN TO ENHANCE & EXTEND YOUR YEARS OVER 40

ELLINGTON DARDEN, PH.D.

A PERIGEE BOOK

A Perigee Book
Published by The Berkley Publishing Group
A division of Penguin Putnam Inc.
375 Hudson Street
New York, NY 10014

First edition: January 1995
Published simultaneously in Canada.

The Penguin Putnam Inc. World Wide Web site address is
http://www.penguinputnam.com

Library of Congress Cataloging-in-Publication Data

Darden, Ellington.
Living longer stronger: the 6-week plan to enhance
& extend your years over 40/Ellington Darden.
p. cm.
"A Perigee Book."
Includes bibliographical references.
ISBN 0-399-51900-9
1. Middle aged men—Health and hygiene.
2. Physical fitness for men.   I. Title.
RA777.8.D37 1995   94-26838
613'.04234—dc20   CIP

Printed in the United States of America

20   19   18   17   16   15   14   13   12   11   10   9   8

This book is printed on acid-free paper.

ILLUSTRATION CREDITS

Gene Bednarek: viii, xiv, 32, 46, 72, 94, 128, 130, 178; Walter Coker: 39, 74; Inge Cook: 44;
Tom Cunningham: 121; Ellington Darden: xii, 2, 8, 11, 15, 132; Paul Hillman: 38, Ken Hutchins: 18;
Kurt Lischka: 199; Chris Lund: 101, 137, 166; Buster O'Connor: 69, 70, 71, 152–164, 180, 188–197;
Rob Singleton: 43, 202; Nellie Wiggins: 96

ACKNOWLEDGMENTS

I acknowledge and thank the following people who made this project successful: John Duff for his editing
and guidance; Terry Duschinski for his research and writing; Jenifer Doherty for her word processing;
Betsy Styron for her comments and ideas; Buster O'Connor for his design; Lee Seabrook for her layout;
Gene Bednarek for his photography; Angela Miller for her agenting skills; Joe Cirulli for his encourage-
ment; and Tim Patterson for his overall support of *Living Longer Stronger*.

WARNING

The routines in this book are intended only for healthy men and women.
People with health problems should not follow these routines without a physician's approval.
Before beginning any exercise or dietary program, always consult with your doctor.

Contents

IV. Relearning Food and Nutrition

V. Removing Excessive Body Fat

VI. Rebuilding and Reducing Programs

VII. REJUVENATING YOUR LIFE

STRAIGHT TALK FROM ELLINGTON DARDEN

I'm going to show you how to maximize the basics.

Your body needs more muscle and less fat.

You are never too out of shape to begin a program of proper exercising and eating.

Everything you require to get started, you probably already own.

Efficient guidelines, combined with appropriate actions, produce positive results in your body.

A physical change that you can see and feel increases your motivation.

Now is the time to commit.

THE LIVING-LONGER-STRONGER CHALLENGE

In only six weeks, you can:

- Reshape your physique by losing 21 pounds of body fat.

- Flatten your belly by eliminating 3½ inches from your waist.

- Harden your arms and chest by building 4 pounds of solid muscle.

- Powerize your back and legs by increasing their strength by 50 percent.

These challenges, as well as others throughout this program, will provide a new appreciation of your muscles. As a result, you'll be well on your way toward the rejuvenation of your body.

A revitalized body will allow you to live a more productive second middle age and beyond.

THE SECOND MIDDLE AGE

In 1900, scientists divided a man's life into three stages: youth, 0–20 years; middle age, 21–40 years; and old age, 41–death. The average man living in the United States at the turn of the century could expect to die at age 47. The prevalent belief then was that a man over 40 could not be productive and creative.

Nearly a century later, an American man's life expectancy is 72 years—and gradually increasing with each new set of statistics. As a result, there's an emerging second middle age.

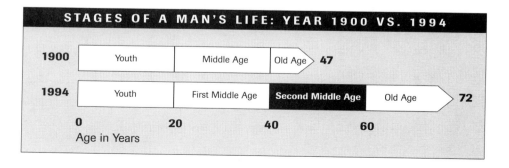

The concept of a second middle age was introduced by Dr. Lydia Bronte in her 1993 book, *The Longevity Factor.* Narrowing her concept to men only, I define this second middle age as a stage of manhood between 40 and 60 that has existed only in recent years.

Dr. Robert Butler, head of geriatric medicine at Mount Sinai Medical School, notes that from 1900 to 1990 average life expectancy grew more than it did in the previous 2,000 years. This is an unprecedented leap forward in longevity. A man celebrating his sixtieth birthday today should be preparing for another two or three decades of creative adulthood. Unfortunately, many men are and remain ill-prepared for this journey.

This second middle age in a man's life is a pivotal time. It's a time to look back, evaluate, learn, apply, and move forward. Restore, retrain, rethink, relearn, rebuild, and renew are the challenges of his fifth and sixth decades.

Successfully dealing with this second middle age enables a man to boldly enter his twilight years—those after age 60—armed with the knowledge of healthy habits. Statistics reveal that most American men die not so much from a particular disease, but from how they choose to live. This book is about distinguishing wise choices from foolish ones.

A MUSCULAR FOUNDATION

The foundation of this book is the research I've been doing since 1965. My studies prove that muscles are the engines of the body. They perform work. They demand energy. They produce movement. They offer protection.

Building stronger muscles is the single best medicine a man can prescribe for himself. Stronger muscles fend off degeneration. Stronger muscles escalate productivity. Stronger muscles are the key to living longer.

In October 1993 I encountered my fiftieth birthday. Twenty-five years ago, 50 sounded old to me. But now, I'm looking forward to another 50 years of vigorous living.

The week after my birthday, I had to present my driver's license as proof that I was 21 years of age to gain entry into a nightclub. This amazed my girlfriend, who is half my age, because the bouncer at the door didn't bother to examine her date of birth. I'll admit it was rather dark in the hallway entrance, which helped to shadow the gray in my hair.

LESSONS IN UNLEARNING

When I was in the first grade at Sam Houston Elementary School in Conroe, Texas, I played the role of the strongman in our annual student play, "At the Circus." Dressed in a leopard-skin shirt, wearing a fake handlebar mustache, and lugging a cardboard barbell that was labeled "500 Pounds," my overhead lift was convincing, at least in my mind. Later, my charade was undone when the tumbler, a girl about half my size, strutted around the stage pushing the barbell effortlessly overhead with only one arm. I got over the embarrassment eventually but never did overcome my fascination with strength.

I was a good athlete in my youth, especially skilled in baseball, football, and basketball. By the time I was 14 and my peers were starting to give me some real competition, I knew I needed an edge to keep pace in the world of teen sports. So, in the summer of 1959, I got my first real barbells and set up my home gym in the garage. I guess I was one of the only boys in high school that practiced strength training seriously—and it showed. In four years my body weight increased from 130 to 205 pounds. My performance in sports improved and I finished high school with 13 letters in four sports. By age 18 I was training 2 hours a day, five or six days a week. It was an obsession.

During my college days at Baylor University, I was inspired by local gym owner Ed Cook to get involved in competitive bodybuilding. During the next five years, I won more than 50 trophies including Mr. Oklahoma and Mr. Texas. In 1968 I entered graduate school at Florida State University and continued to train and participate in contests across the South, collecting another 50 trophies and finally winning the Collegiate Mr. America.

I had spent thousands of hours training; training that I considered invaluable. But now, more than 20 years later, I know that I could have produced much better results in a fraction of the time. And I could have accomplished these goals without the pulled biceps, torn deltoids, lower back problems, and sprained knee ligaments.

When I was 28 and about to finish my Ph.D. program in exercise science, I met Arthur Jones, the founder of Nautilus. Jones confronted me with the following: "If you can unlearn everything you've learned about exercise—and you can do this unlearning before you reach 40—you'll be headed in the right direction. Then maybe you can learn something of value."

It took me a dozen years to unlearn what I thought I knew about exercise and strength training. In the years since my fortieth birthday, I've discovered a great deal more from the wisdom of individuals like Arthur Jones and through working with thousands of people of every age and condition who desire to be physically fit.

"Success comes from good judgment," Jones says. "Good judgment comes from experience. Experience comes from bad judgment." In other words, you have to make mistakes to learn. And while I don't think that I can completely overcome human nature, I hope that the advice and guidance in this book will help you profit from my unlearning process, avoid the most critical mistakes, and achieve your goal to live longer stronger.

SUCCESS STORY: ZACK TANNERY, AGE 50

- Lost 28½ pounds of fat
- Built 6 pounds of muscle
- Trimmed 4 inches off his waist in 42 days.

"The program simply changed my life. I feel like a new man. Most of my aches and pains no longer bother me."

Today, my waistline is smaller than it was 25 years ago, and so is my percentage of body fat. My strength and muscle mass are still at high levels. My resting heart rate is 54 beats per minute. Obviously, I do practice what I recommend.

The oldest members of the post-World War II generation, the baby boomers, will also soon turn 50. Not only do some of them deny being over the hill, but many are planning new careers, broadening their horizons with different challenges.

To meet these challenges, *Living Longer Stronger* is valuable reading for every baby boomer.

For more than 30 years I've been actively involved in strength training and bodybuilding. Bodybuilding may bring to your mind the image of oiled bodies in tiny posing trunks flexing their muscles. Yes, competitive bodybuilding does require a good bit of muscular display. The type of bodybuilding and strength training that I'm referring to in this course, however, entails developing your muscles for performance, leanness, and fitness.

STEP-BY-STEP PROGRESSION

Each of the 43 chapters in this book supplies easy-to-apply guidelines on living a stronger, leaner, longer, and more fruitful life. By incorporating these guidelines into an effective plan, which is outlined in Part VI, you'll reduce your body fat, flatten your stomach, muscularize your arms and chest, strengthen your legs, and improve your heart-lung endurance in only six weeks. You'll be amazed with your new body and your new outlook on your second middle age. Soon you'll be in possession of the greatest reward of all: time, more productive time.

Welcome to *Living Longer Stronger*.

That's exactly what you're going to accomplish!

Ellington Darden, Ph.D.
Gainesville, Florida

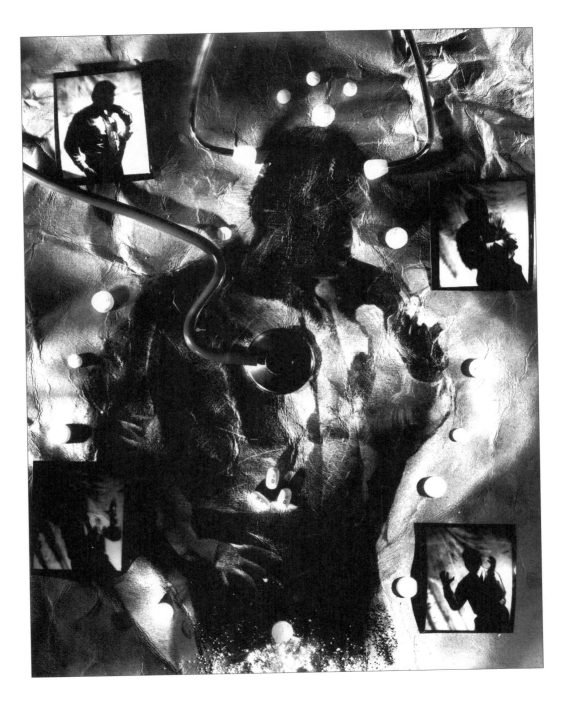

I.
RESOLVING AGE-OLD PROBLEMS

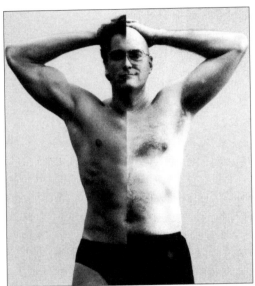

*Blake Boyd, 23, and his father Bill Boyd, 52, have prac-
ticed proper strength training for many years. Keeping
the muscles strong combats much of the decline in a
man's health as he gets older.*

1

AGING, BIOMARKERS, AND STRENGTH

Aging is too commonly associated with weakness, wrinkles, gray hair, retirement, forgetfulness, frailty, nursing homes, and death. Our concepts about age result from a complex mixture of prejudices, expectations, customs, and even legislation.

To better understand these concepts, scientists have targeted the aging process for detailed study. Although much research is yet to be done, there are still exciting findings to share.

Erosion of the human body is not inevitable, conclude many scientific reports. Only death is unavoidable. Barring disease, many body functions decline very slowly if engaged in proper exercise, nutrition, stimulation, and support.

The focus in this book is on rebuilding and maintaining strength, health, independence, and vitality for the longest possible time. To a great extent, you can control your own destiny.

BIOMARKERS INTERVENTION

In their 1991 book, *Biomarkers: The 10 Determinants of Aging You Can Control*, Dr. William Evans and Dr. Irwin Rosenberg report the findings of studies at the U.S. Department of Agriculture Human Nutrition Research Center on Aging at Tufts University. Their ten biomarkers, or physiological factors associated with aging, are as follows:

1. Muscle mass
2. Strength
3. Basal metabolic rate
4. Body fat percentage
5. Aerobic capacity
6. Blood-sugar tolerance

7. Cholesterol/HDL ratio

8. Blood pressure

9. Bone density

10. The body's ability to regulate its internal temperature

THE POWER OF STRENGTH TRAINING

Not surprising to me is that each of these biomarkers is improved through the type of exercise recommended in *Living Longer Stronger*. This type of exercise was called weightlifting 40 years ago. Later it was modified to weight training, strength training, and progressive resistance exercise. Then the concept, with the media's help, came to be known as pumping iron. Although all of these concepts apply, in my books and writings I've always been partial to *strength training*. Strength training is also one of the keys to successful muscle building.

The Living-Longer-Stronger version of strength training is somewhat different from what you may have done in the past. It involves the lifting and lowering of weights (barbells, dumbbells, and machines), but each exercise requires a specific style. That specific style features slow, smooth movement. Slow and smooth movement, which eliminates excessive momentum, as opposed to fast and jerky motion, is much more productive at stimulating your muscles to grow larger and stronger. You'll learn more about this style in later chapters.

Briefly, here's how proper strength training affects each biomarker.

Both (1) muscle mass and (2) strength go together. As your body adapts and lifts heavier and heavier weights, your muscles get stronger and larger. An average man, through proper strength training, can expect to increase his overall strength by 5 percent per week. Consequently, this 5 percent strength increase will add approximately one-half pound of muscle to his body.

Additional muscle elevates your (3) basal metabolic rate. Given that your dietary calories per day remain unchanged, you'll notice a slight reduction in your (4) body fat percentage.

Proper strength training can boost your (5) aerobic capacity by improving your heart's ability to pump oxygen-rich blood to the working muscles.

Your (6) blood-sugar tolerance, or your body's ability to control the level of sugar in the blood, is enhanced by strength training. Generally, as a man gets older, he gradually loses muscle and gains fat. As a result, he needs more insulin—

THEORIES OF AGING

From among the many theories that explain aging, here are some of the more popular:

- Your cells contain a built-in genetic program that sets the pace of aging and determines the outer limit of your life span.

- Your body provides a fixed amount of energy that gradually shrinks over time until it's finally used up.

- Aging is the result of a gradual deterioration of the immune system, which makes your body more susceptible to infection and disease.

- Free radicals, molecules with unpaired electrons, exist normally in your body, but they are also produced by tobacco smoke, air pollution, the sun, burned foods, and certain drugs. In the presence of oxygen, free radicals trigger a chain reaction that causes cells to deteriorate in a similar way as exposure to salt air causes metal to rust.

- A gland, possibly the pituitary, secretes a death hormone. This death hormone in turn trips the aging process and eventually ends your life.

- Your cells supply the seeds of their own destruction. Scientists have succeeded in growing certain cells indefinitely in a laboratory culture. Investigating these seemingly immortal cells, the researchers found that all of them lacked a specific human chromosome. When the missing chromosome was placed in the cells, they began to age.

a hormone that removes sugar from the blood and transfers it to the body's tissues for fuel. Added muscle decreases the need for insulin, and helps prevent adult-onset diabetes.

Several studies show that strength training and lowering body fat can raise blood levels of protective high-density lipoprotein (HDL) cholesterol. Plus, total cholesterol can decrease. The (7) cholesterol/HDL ratio often significantly improves—which is an important factor in preventing heart attacks.

Along with controlling blood cholesterol, the exercise programs recommended in this book can help regulate (8) blood pressure. Learning to lift and lower heavy weights in the correct manner, however, is instrumental in getting the best possible results and avoiding some of the related problems. You'll get the most up-to-date instruction on how to do this in Chapter 13.

Any time you build a muscle larger and stronger, you correspondingly increase your (9) bone density. Bone thinning, or osteoporosis, can be warded off with proper strength exercise.

Finally, strength training improves (10) the body's ability to regulate its internal temperature. Your body comes with a built-in thermostat, which requires plenty of water to function correctly. Since your muscles are mostly composed of water, the six-week plan described in Part VI of this book promotes the drinking of at least one gallon of water each day. Plus, having more muscle on your body means you'll have a higher total water content, which helps regulate your internal temperature as well.

SAY YES TO THE LIVING-LONGER-STRONGER PLAN

Can a 40-, 50-, or 60-year-old man who hasn't been physically active for years really forge into this program and expect to hold back or even reverse his biomarkers' decline? Yes! And will doing so reverse his body's aging? Yes, again!

Throughout this book I'll present plenty of evidence to back up what I'm saying.

2
EASY-CHAIR ATROPHY

As the average man ages, he loses muscle and gets weaker.

After their teenage years, most men become less active with each passing decade. With the advent of labor-saving devices, many tasks once performed manually are now executed at the flick of a switch.

Even our leisure activities have been altered by technology. When was the last time you enjoyed a Sunday outing? A row on a lake? A walk in the woods? Thanks to the NFL, the NBA, the PGA, and other perks of cable and commercial TV, there is hardly reason to leave our air-conditioned dens.

Our quantum leap in technology has resulted in a steady decline of physiology. The physical demands of everyday living are simply not what they used to be. We're living longer because of better medicine. But living *even* longer stronger requires investment in the vibrant health habits that this book is about.

BREAKDOWN OF MUSCLE

Research by Dr. Gilbert Forbes of the University of Rochester School of Medicine shows that the average man loses a half-pound of muscle per year between the ages of 20 and 50. This average man is one who does not engage in regular strength-building exercise. As a 50-year-old, his body is 15 pounds less muscular than at age 20.

The loss of muscle and strength—and thus probable decline in other biomarkers—is strictly from a lack of use. Sooner or later, this disuse is likely to manifest itself in a physical ailment such as a heart attack, arthritis, or a degenerative disk. From there, it's usually a steady downward spiral.

Strength may not be a panacea, but, of all the factors over which you have some control, it is a critical one. Many of the aches and pains of old age can be averted. It is important that you understand the perils of ignoring muscle.

Atrophy, the shrinkage of muscle tissue from disuse, involves metabolic breakdown of muscle into its constituent compounds, which are removed by the bloodstream.

Atrophied muscle does not turn into fat. Muscle and fat are composed of different cells, and it's impossible to turn one into the other.

Muscle cells that atrophy simply lose their fluids, become smaller and weaker, and lessen their ability to contract.

LESS HORSEPOWER

Muscles are the engines of the body; weaker muscles mean less horsepower, and a marked decline in performance results.

If you ever fractured a limb and spent several weeks in a cast, you will have experienced a rapid atrophying of muscles from total immobility, along with accompanying pain in the joints.

Without proper strength training, many of us place our entire bodies into a cast of sedentary living. The effects progress more slowly than what we experience with a fractured arm, but the results are just as damaging.

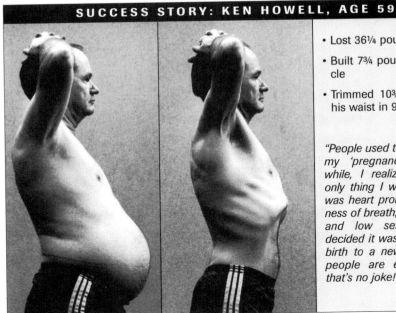

SUCCESS STORY: KEN HOWELL, AGE 59

- Lost 36¼ pounds of fat
- Built 7¾ pounds of muscle
- Trimmed 10¾ inches off his waist in 96 days.

"People used to joke about my 'pregnancy.' After a while, I realized that the only thing I was expecting was heart problems, shortness of breath, a sore back, and low self-esteem. I decided it was time to give birth to a new body. Now people are envious, and that's no joke!"

FUEL OF HIGH ACHIEVEMENT

Recent findings from *Club Business International* reveal that more than twice as many chief executive officers of major corporations exercise on a regular basis compared to adult men in general.

Do CEOs exercise because they are high achievers? Are they high achievers because they exercise? While there are no exact answers, one plausible theory is that the discipline of regular exercise, as well as its effect on health and vigor, contributes to the achievement of lofty goals.

In addition to labor-saving devices, modern technology has provided efficient exercise tools and useful information that enable proper strength training to be achieved in as little as three 20-minute workouts per week. You don't have to be a gym rat, a musclehead, or a fitness fanatic. In the same amount of time that you commit to everyday hygiene, you can factor effective exercise into your daily life.

Strength training is an integral element of productive living. Time invested in averting Easy-Chair Atrophy pays bonus dividends that mature during the second middle age.

3

CREEPING OBESITY

While a man's body is losing a half-pound of muscle, on average, each year between ages 20 and 50, his fat cells are thriving. The fat-cell phenomenon progresses at three times the rate of muscle loss—only it's a gain, not a reduction. As far as your health and vitality are concerned, these phenomena are both moving in a negative direction.

So slowly are these dual changes occurring that often it takes a decade or more to notice that something major is happening to your body.

FAT GAIN

The average man between the ages of 20 and 50 gains 1.5 pounds of fat each year. That adds up to 15 pounds of fat gain per decade or 45 pounds in 30 years. This slow gain of body fat is what nutritionists call creeping obesity.

Actually, this creeping obesity is somewhat disguised by the shrinking of muscle mass that is going on at the same time. A 15-pound muscle loss means that the overall gain in body weight is 30 pounds, not 45. In fact, the loss of muscle compounds the situation. Here's why.

RESTING METABOLIC RATE

A person's resting metabolic rate is the number of calories that his body requires to function in a relaxed, resting state. The brain and internal organs such as the heart, lungs, liver, and kidneys, require a lot of energy. But it's the skeletal muscles, which comprise from 35 to 50 percent of a man's body weight, that have the most energy potential.

Add a pound of muscle to a man's body, and his resting metabolic rate goes up approximately 50 calories per day. The inverse is also notable. Lose a pound of muscle through disuse atrophy, and the rate is lowered by 50 calories per day.

Interestingly, fat also has a metabolic rate: approximately 2 calories per pound per day. Muscle is twenty-five times as active metabolically as the same amount of fat.

You've probably noticed that it is more difficult to shed excess fat than it used to be. Long-term metabolism studies reveal that an average man experiences a 0.5 percent reduction in resting metabolic rate each year between 20 and 50 years of age. The gradual loss of muscle mass each year is primarily responsible for this metabolic slowdown.

MUSCLE YOUR FAT AWAY

Certainly, controlling dietary calories is an important aspect of combating creeping obesity. But equally important is the building, or rebuilding, of muscle mass.

Do not let your fat cells grow while your muscles wither. It's time to muscle your fat away.

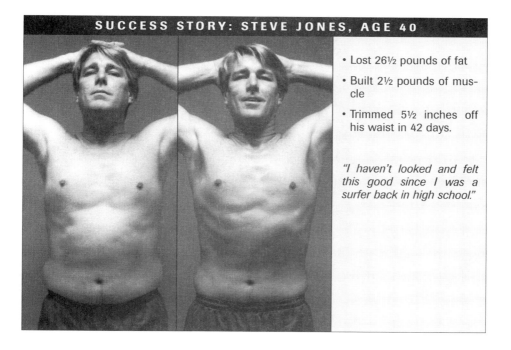

SUCCESS STORY: STEVE JONES, AGE 40

- Lost 26½ pounds of fat
- Built 2½ pounds of muscle
- Trimmed 5½ inches off his waist in 42 days.

"I haven't looked and felt this good since I was a surfer back in high school."

THE GOOD LIFE

I sincerely want the information and program in this book to help you look younger, feel better, and live longer. In fact, if you accomplish these goals, doing so will help me look younger, feel better, and live longer.

How can this happen?

As the life expectancy of people increases, the total storehouse of knowledge and experience automatically expands. That expansion of knowledge and experience enhances the good life for everyone.

Ben Douglas, in his book *AgeLess*, makes a convincing argument for the relationship between increasing life expectancy and improving problem-solving ability.

"The whole process," Douglas says, "is self-perpetuating. As we solve more problems, we will live longer, and as we live longer we will be able to solve more problems."

The drawing below illustrates this concept.

Let's consider 100,000 people in two different situations. First, the people develop into adults, are educated and skilled in a profession, and start using their talents at age 25. Gradually, their numbers decrease as a result of typical accidents and diseases. The survivors use their skills until age 65 and then retire. Thus, the darker shaded area under the curve represents the contribution of the body of knowledge and experience of the original 100,000 people.

In the second situation, the individuals are much more prevention-minded. As deaths from diseases and accidents decrease, more people live productively to near the end of the human life span of 115 years. The amount of knowledge and experience that is gained is shown by the lighter-shaded area under the curve. This lighter-shaded area represents a new pool of knowledge and experience, which will provide increased potential for problem-solving.

Sometime in the twenty-first century, we'll have a problem-solving potential in the United States that will be similar to the second situation. When this happens, we'll see dramatic changes in all aspects of our lives. It will indeed be a good life.

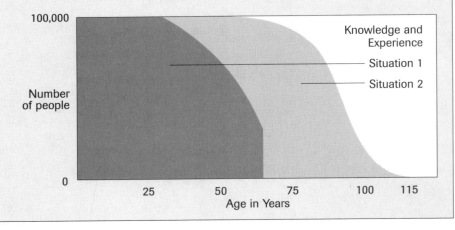

4

BUILDING MUSCLE AND LOSING FAT . . . SIMULTANEOUSLY

Although at first glance this chapter title may sound like one of those questionable advertisements you see in muscle magazines, it's absolutely accurate. With the Living-Longer-Stronger eating and exercising plan you can build muscle and lose fat at the same time.

LOSING AND BUILDING

The average man I've trained over the years is 6 feet tall and weighs 175 pounds at age 20. His body is composed of 12 percent bone, 15 percent fat, 47 percent muscle, and 26 percent organs, skin, and other.

Using the statistics from the last two chapters, let's fast-forward 20 years.

At age 40, our average man has lost 10 pounds of muscle and gained 30 pounds of fat. His percentage of body fat has gone from 15 to 28.85, and his muscle has decreased from 47 to 37.05 percent. As a result, his body weight has risen from 175 to 195.

In 20 years, our average man has gone from a fairly decent physical condition to being overfat, undermuscled, and out of shape. Furthermore, he is now at

	HOW THE AVERAGE MAN LOSES AND GAINS					
	Age 20		Age 40		After Six Weeks of Living Longer Stronger	
	Percent	Pounds	Percent	Pounds	Percent	Pounds
Bone	12.00	21.00	10.77	21.00	11.80	21.00
Fat	15.00	26.25	28.85	56.25	19.80	35.25
Muscle	47.00	82.25	37.05	72.25	42.84	76.25
Organs, Skin, Other	26.00	45.50	23.33	45.50	25.56	45.50
		175.00		195.00		178.00

higher risk for specific medical conditions, such as high blood pressure, kidney disease, diabetes mellitus, stroke, and impairment of heart function.

IN ONLY SIX WEEKS

What our average man needs is the Living-Longer-Stronger plan that is described in Part VI. In only six weeks, he can lose 21 pounds of fat while simultaneously building 4 pounds of muscle. As a result, his body fat percentage will decrease from 28.85 to 19.80 and his muscle will increase from 37.05 to 42.84 percent.

Although he has not quite recaptured his 20-year-old body, he is close. If he continues the program for another six weeks, his 40-something physique will be in better shape than it was 20 years earlier. And his risks for the listed medical conditions will be significantly reduced.

A FEW EXAMPLES

In my programs over the last few years, I've seen some amazing results occur. For example:

- Michael Brown, a 42-year-old sportscaster, lost 24½ pounds of fat and built 5¼ pounds of muscle in 32 days.

- Richard Ives, a 47-year-old businessman, lost 24¾ pounds of fat and built 4 pounds of muscle in 32 days.

- Ron Travis, a 46-year-old businessman, lost 21¾ pounds of fat and built 5 pounds of muscle in 32 days.

- Jay Bobbitt, a 40-year-old realtor, lost 44½ pounds of fat and built 4 pounds of muscle in 64 days.

- Ted Blake, a 41-year-old plumber, lost 42½ pounds of fat and built 3½ pounds of muscle in 70 days.

- Stephen Peterson, a 40-year-old service manager, lost 42 pounds of fat and built 3½ pounds of muscle in 70 days.

- Doyle Linderman, a 57-year-old postal clerk, lost 32¾ pounds of fat and built 4½ pounds of muscle in 70 days.

- Jim Owens, a 50-year-old businessman, lost 30 pounds of fat and built 4 pounds of muscle in 42 days.

BUILDING FROM FAT

How does your body build muscle on a lower-calorie diet? It draws most of the chemicals necessary for growth from your fat cells. Since a pound of fat supplies 3,500 calories and a pound of muscle contains only 600 calories, it's possible to build 5 pounds of muscle from 1 pound of fat. Over 70 percent of muscle is water, and water is void of calories. Fat, on the other hand, is mostly fat—which is composed of greasy, waxy, lipid material.

One more additional fact about fat and muscle will be of interest to you. Scientists have taken samples of fat and muscle from throughout the human body and actually counted the number of cells. Although this research is still in its infancy and depends on extrapolation, the average man appears to have approximately 25 billion fat cells and 10 billion muscle cells.

Each of these microscopically small cells has the capacity to inflate, like a balloon, or deflate. Obviously, it is to your advantage to inflate your muscle cells and deflate your fat cells.

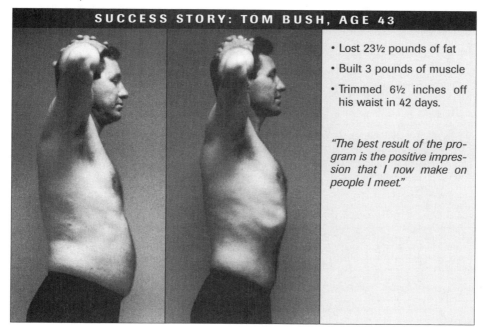

SUCCESS STORY: TOM BUSH, AGE 43

- Lost 23½ pounds of fat
- Built 3 pounds of muscle
- Trimmed 6½ inches off his waist in 42 days.

"The best result of the program is the positive impression that I now make on people I meet."

TO EXPECT

On average, what can a man in his second middle age—between 40 and ~~ect~~ from the recommended Living-Longer-Stronger, strength-training ? He can anticipate the following:

- A 5-percent increase in strength per week, or at least per two weeks, in all the basic exercises. For example, if you can perform the standing biceps curl with a 50-pound barbell for 10 repetitions during week one, then during week two, you should be able to do the same number of repetitions with 52½ pounds. At the end of six weeks, you should be able to curl 65 pounds for 10 repetitions, which translates to a 30-percent improvement in your biceps' strength.

- A ½-pound overall body gain of muscle mass per week. My testing and experience over the years have shown that the average 40- to 60-year-old man can build 3 to 4 pounds of muscle during his initial six-week strength-training program.

The typical 40- to 60-year-old man can continue his strength and muscle mass increases for another six to twelve weeks. Naturally, the rate of gain decreases with progress. But the man who is consistent with the discipline can expect to double his muscular strength and add 10 to 12 pounds of muscle to his body during the first nine to twelve months.

Combine this predicted muscle with a 20- to 40-pound loss of fat, and your own mother may not recognize you at first glance.

Yes, you can build muscle and lose fat—and you can do both simultaneously.

5

WHY MUSCLE MATTERS MOST

It doesn't take an NFL linebacker to operate the TV remote control, press the garage-door opener, navigate a mouse through a computer program, drive a fully automated automobile, or utilize any of the conveniences that fashion our everyday lives. Aside from athletes, bricklayers, and lumberjacks, who, then, requires muscular strength to cope with life at the end of the twentieth century?

The answer is an unequivocal *everyone*. And the older you are, the more crucial it may be.

The size and strength of the muscles is a major factor in determining an individual's body contour. The cosmetic effect should not be underestimated, because how the body looks, in many people's minds, is the motivation behind a fitness regimen. But what doesn't readily meet the eye makes even a stronger case for muscle.

STRENGTH'S SUPERIORITY

Strength is the basis of all physical capability. It is what enables us to defy gravity and stand upright. Strength performs the work of carrying luggage, turning a wrench, bounding up stairs, or pulling an item off a high shelf. In short, muscle strength constantly contributes to our well-being, or the lack of it constitutes a musculoskeletal hazard.

Muscles are where energy is released, where power is produced, and where movement originates. In addition to being the engines of the body, muscles are also shock absorbers. Strength enhances the integrity of the joints, guarding against painful tears in the connective tissues of the knees, neck, shoulders, elbows, ankles and—above all—the lower back.

According to Dr. Jennifer Kelsey of the Yale University School of Medicine and Dr. Augustus White of the Harvard Medical School, 80 percent of men in their second middle age will suffer from lower back pain. These sufferers will spend billions of dollars annually seeking relief for their problems. Strengthening the muscles surrounding the lumbar spine is an important component in both the rehabilitation and prevention of lower back pain.

Aging and Inactivity

"Much of what we call aging," explains Dr. William Evans, coauthor of *Biomarkers*, "is nothing more than the accumulation of a lifetime of inactivity. Muscles shrink. Body fat increases. The results are an increased risk of diabetes, hypertension, and osteoporosis. By preserving muscle mass, we can prevent these problems from occurring."

Of the usual problems associated with aging, Dr. Evans contends, "it's changes in muscle mass that may trigger all of the other changes."

Building a sheath of protective, well-toned muscle can limit risks from minor mishaps. Strength can also help prevent many chronic aches and pains. According to Dr. Vert Mooney, professor of orthopedic surgery at the University of California School of Medicine at San Diego, "Most chronic musculoskeletal pain problems are as a result of a weak link about a joint in the spine, arms, or legs. This weak link is in the soft tissues [meaning muscle and connective tissue]."

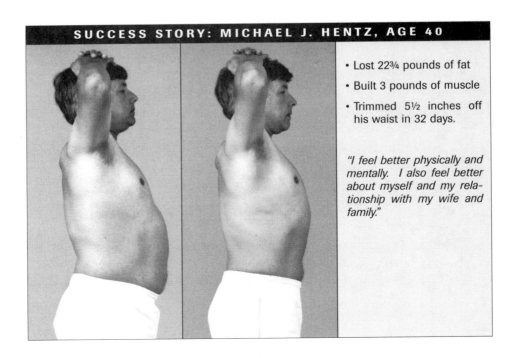

SUCCESS STORY: MICHAEL J. HENTZ, AGE 40

- Lost 22¾ pounds of fat
- Built 3 pounds of muscle
- Trimmed 5½ inches off his waist in 32 days.

"I feel better physically and mentally. I also feel better about myself and my relationship with my wife and family."

Strength training is even a heart-saver. Well-trained leg muscles make it easier to race through airport terminals; muscular arms and back take the strain out of shoveling snow or working in the yard. The less stressful these exertions are, the lower the risk that they'll overstress the heart.

ADAPTING TO DEMANDS, PROGRESSIVELY

For technical purposes, muscular strength is the maximum amount of force that can be exerted by a muscle or muscle group. Your strength is developed through the specific adaptation of your body to imposed demands. This is known as the overload principle. The overloading must be applied in progressive increments. This stimulation, as you will read much more about in later chapters, makes you stronger.

But strength training, performed properly, doesn't stop at muscular development.

6

NOT JUST STRONGER BUT ENDURING, AND FLEXIBLE

The established triad of well-rounded fitness is muscular strength, cardiovascular endurance, and joint flexibility. The objective of *Living Longer Stronger*, and the program I've devised to achieve it, incorporate these components into one potent package.

There is no need for multiple programs. In the past this book might have matriculated from handwritten manuscript, to typewriter, to typesetter, and then to plates for the printing press. Now there's a computer that rolls virtually all those steps into one operation. Our exercise technology has likewise advanced to the point of time-saving efficiency.

Examine these fringe benefits of the strength-building strategy of the Living-Longer-Stronger program.

CARDIOVASCULAR ENDURANCE

Your cardiovascular system is comprised of the heart, arteries, capillaries, and veins. Your heart is a special four-chambered muscle that serves as a storage tank and a pump for moving blood through your body. Arteries are the tubular vessels that carry blood away from your heart. Capillaries are tiny single-layer vessels in the tissues themselves where the actual exchange of oxygen, nutrients, and waste materials takes place. Your capillaries then connect with a system of small veins, which gradually become larger as they return blood to your heart for recirculation.

Improving cardiovascular endurance requires:

• That the exercise must be hard enough to elevate your heart rate to 60 to 85 percent of its maximum beats per minute.

• Your elevated heart rate must be sustained for a minimum of 10 minutes.

• Such exercise should be repeated at least three times a week.

Estimate your maximum heart rate by subtracting your age from 220. If you are 50, your estimated maximum heart rate is 220 minus 50, or 170 beats per minute. For cardiovascular endurance, your workout should enable you to maintain a heart rate of 60 to 85 percent of your maximum, or 102 to 144 beats per minute.

STRENGTH AND CARDIOVASCULAR ENDURANCE

Typically we think of jogging, swimming, stair-climbing, and cycling as activities for improving cardiovascular endurance. This is true, but a well-devised strength-training workout produces cardiovascular stimulation as well as muscle gain and joint flexibility.

Because it does not matter to your heart which muscles are being exercised to elevate your heart rate to the desired level, working your arms has exactly the same effect on your heart as exercise involving your legs, provided the total amount of work and the pace are the same.

A strength-training workout can maintain an elevated heart rate so long as the rest between exercises is minimal: usually 15 to 30 seconds. Your workout should be organized into a sequence of exercises that you initiate one right after another. This style of training is similar to the no-huddle offense you now see in professional football. In other words, after each exercise, get to the next one as if time were running out.

By maintaining an elevated heart rate, a no-huddle circuit of strength training provides improvement in cardiovascular endurance, along with increased strength.

JOINT FLEXIBILITY

Flexibility is being able to bend forward while keeping your legs stiff and touch your toes. It is being able to reach behind your back, turn your head, or stretch comfortably into an assortment of positions. Most of us second middle-agers remember a game called Twister. Some time in the past we probably also shimmied under a bamboo pole in a dance called the Limbo.

Flexibility is the range and ease of movement of a body part around a joint. How much you are able to stretch is essential to the maintenance and safekeeping of joints, muscles, and connective tissues. Anatomically, the limiting factors in flexibility are tendons, ligaments, muscle fibers, and muscle fascia or sheath. Tendons are not meant to be stretched. Ligaments adapt to slight stretching but once stretched will not return to normal length. Muscle fibers have great capacity for stretching. The muscle fascia is a stretchable connective tissue sheath enclosing the muscle fibers.

Through adaptation resulting from proper exercise, muscle and muscle fascia will stretch and become more flexible.

FULL-RANGE STRENGTH AND FLEXIBILITY

The adaptation process that produces enhanced flexibility requires stretching into a position beyond the normal range of movement for a particular limb. Stretching needs to be done smoothly—never by a sudden force or a jerk.

Stretching also needs to take place in a situation that I call *under load*. This means that the targeted muscle must not only be stretched, but also must be challenged to lift a weight that is heavy for it. This under-load stretching is applied through full-range, progressive, strength-training exercises. The full-range element of it—from a point of maximum stretch moving into full-muscular contraction—qualifies the endeavor to also be termed flexibility training.

A POTENT PACKAGE

I used to *not* know better. I used to believe that it was necessary to have separate routines for muscular strength, cardiovascular endurance, and joint flexibility. I now know that these separate routines are wasteful and inefficient.

Living Longer Stronger, therefore, acknowledges muscular strength as the central factor of fitness and promotes strength training as the best form of exercise. Proper strength training is indeed a potent package.

7
What About Aerobics?

On my frequent two-block walks between my town house and my office at the Gainesville (Florida) Health & Fitness Center, along the street I encounter numerous runners subjecting their lower bodies to unsuspected and potentially dangerous impact forces. Then as I enter the fitness center, I'm engulfed by the aerobics people using computerized cycling machines or stair-climbing machines, or engaged in dance classes.

These runners, cyclists, stair-climbers, and dancers are presumably trying to sustain their target heart rates to achieve their fitness goals, evidently unaware that far superior conditioning is afforded by the center's 150 strength-training machines of various types and a complete free-weight room, all of which is also heavily utilized.

ADVENTURES IN AEROBICS

In 1968, Dr. Kenneth Cooper published *Aerobics*, which became a bestseller and a trendsetter. Cooper defined aerobics as large-muscle, endurance-type activities that increased involvement of the heart and lungs for a prolonged time. Furthermore, he evaluated and ranked various activities that met his aerobic criteria. Cross-country skiing, swimming, and running were at the top, followed by cycling and walking. Strength training, by the way, was ranked near the bottom.

What is the genesis of the term *aerobics*? Before Cooper's first book, *aerobic* was used as an adjective and meant "living in oxygen." Certain bacteria that live and grow in oxygen are called aerobes.

Cooper, however, used *aerobics* as a noun to refer to his rated activities and point system. Initially, as he tells the story, he had chosen a more conventional title for the concept and book. But the publisher talked him into changing it at the last minute because the word *aerobics* was more intriguing.

Several years later, aerobic was attached to dancing by Jacki Sorensen. Soon, aerobic-dancing studios began to spring up throughout the United States.

But it wasn't until the 1980s that aerobics really swept the country. It did so as a result of Jane Fonda and her videotapes. Kathy Smith and other women followed in Fonda's trail. Fun and popular music were emphasized in most of these aerobic-dancing programs.

In 1985, the majority of the people in this country believed that aerobics implied only aerobic dancing. Today, with the arrival of stair-climbing machines, step classes, computerized cycling machines, rowers, and treadmills, cross-training machines, plus dozens of glitzy fitness videotapes, there is an association in most people's minds back to Cooper's original meaning of the word.

In fact, the 1989 edition of *The Oxford English Dictionary* defined *aerobics* as: "physical exercise for producing beneficial changes in the respiratory and circulatory system by activities which require only a modest increase of oxygen intake and so can be maintained."

Do you need some element of aerobics to have a well-rounded fitness program? I could give you a ten-thousand-word explanation, but the bottom line is that by letting no more than 15 to 30 seconds elapse from one strength exercise to the next, and training at a high-intensity level, you're receiving significant aerobic benefit.

I'll concentrate here on telling you why this is commonly misunderstood.

STEREOTYPING STRENGTH TRAINING

When Dr. Kenneth Cooper and his colleagues initially studied the cardiovascular effects of various activities, they tested bodybuilders and weightlifters who had been trained in the traditional manner. This traditional manner consisted of 15 seconds of explosive-type lifting followed by a several-minute rest period. They might continue these lifting-resting cycles for more than an hour. The heart and lungs of such subjects are not receiving the steady pace of work required for cardiovascular benefits. So, naturally, these traditionally trained bodybuilders and weightlifters performed near the bottom on endurance-type tests.

Thus, a stereotype—that strength training provided poor aerobic or cardiovascular conditioning—was established in 1968.

Almost anyone who strength trains with short rest periods between exercises knows better. I was a subject in an unpublished cardiovascular study at Florida State University in 1969 that involved a circuit of barbell exercises. My heart rate and oxygen consumption were monitored throughout the workout. They were both in the range required to elicit positive benefits for my heart and lungs.

The first few times I trained on a complete line of Nautilus equipment in 1970, even though I wasn't measured on any parameter, I felt an even greater response from my cardiovascular system. In fact, over the next three or four years, I trained hundreds of people on Nautilus equipment who experienced similar effects. But we still didn't have objective data. All we had were subjective experiences.

In 1975 Nautilus Sports/Medical Industries and the United States Military Academy at West Point, New York, combined forces for a joint research project. Under the direction of Dr. James A. Peterson, I helped to strength-train 20 varsity football players for six weeks. In only 17 workouts averaging less than 30 minutes each, these men increased their strength an average of 59 percent. They improved their cardiovascular endurance so much that they reduced their times for the two-mile run by an average of 88 seconds.

The critics noted, however, that maximal oxygen uptake was not used as a measure of cardiorespiratory fitness. So, they questioned the validity of the results.

Finally, a strength-training study

> ### INJURIES—A LITTLE UNDERSTOOD PROBLEM
>
> More than 20 million injuries are sustained each year in the United States as a result of sports and fitness activities. To put this number in perspective, 20 million is more injuries than the people of our country have suffered in all our wars to date.
>
> Which activities are the most dangerous? There's an 86 percent probability of being injured each year if you play tackle football. That's self-evident because football is a combative sport. At 83 percent is gymnastics, which seems unjustified until you understand the very high forces involved and the great flexibility required to do many of the competitive events. Following at 80 percent is the popular aerobic activity, jogging or running.
>
> In the top ten also is aerobic dancing. At one time, in the high-impact years, aerobic dancing was at the 70-percent level of injury. Introducing the low-impact style lowered it to the mid-40 percent level. But with the arrival of step classes and the return of high-impact dancing, now called high-energy in many places, the numbers are moving back toward 70 percent.

reported in a 1985 issue of the *Research Quarterly for Exercise and Sport* did include maximal oxygen uptake. Dr. Stephen Messier and Mary Dill of Wake Forest University measured the aerobic conditioning benefits of 36 male college students divided into three groups: those training on Nautilus equipment, those lifting free weights in the traditional style, and those engaged in a running program. All subjects trained three times per week for ten weeks.

The results showed the Nautilus trainees enjoyed the same aerobic benefits that the runners did. They both improved in maximal oxygen uptake by more than 10 percent. Furthermore, the running group trained 50 percent longer than the

Nautilus group: 30 minutes per session compared to 20 minutes per session. The group that exercised in the traditional lifting fashion actually performed slightly worse in cardiovascular tests at the end than at the beginning.

Only when the rest periods between strength-training exercises are in the 15- to 30-second range can the elevated heart rate and oxygen consumption be sustained for maximum aerobic benefits. And, once again, training your muscles and your heart at the same time is more efficient, effective, and much safer.

It's time for the stereotype—that strength training provides poor aerobic conditioning—to be relegated to the past.

> ### EXAMPLE OF NAUTILUS CIRCUIT USED IN WAKE FOREST STUDY
>
> 1. Hip & Back
> 2. Compound Leg*
>   a. Leg Extension
>   b. Leg Press
> 3. Leg Curl
> 4. Pullover/Torso Arm*
>   a. Pullover
>   b. Pulldown
> 5. Double Chest*
>   a. Arm Cross
>   b. Decline Press
> 6. Double Shoulder*
>   a. Lateral Raise
>   b. Overhead Press
> 7. Biceps Curl
> 8. Triceps Extension
>
> *Dual exercise machine

MUSCLES FOR FAT BURNING

Another aerobics-related fallacy is the idea that to shed body fat, you must train aerobically. This is believed because aerobic activity, or low-intensity exercise, generally burns fat as fuel. Strength training, or high-intensity exercise, basically utilizes carbohydrate energy. Recent research by Dr. Douglas Ballor of the University of Wisconsin reveals that the type of fuel burned during energy production is replaced during and after the exercise by foods eaten, stored carbohydrates, and stored fats.

No matter which energy system your body uses, it burns calories. More than any single factor in fat loss, calories count: dietary calories, exercise calories, and metabolic rate calories.

You will make much better use of your time by stimulating growth of your muscles—muscles that will burn extra calories while at rest the next day. That is the awesome calorie-burning advantage of strength-building workouts.

NO AEROBICS ADDED, BUT . . .

A half-hour of stair-climbing, cycling, running, or dancing won't provide near the fitness benefits of a circuit of high-intensity strength training. Still, there are men who will insist on their computerized aerobic exercise. Perhaps it is because the electronic displays on such machines provide feedback: zipping through rows of lights is kind of like checking off items on a to-do list.

The Living-Longer-Stronger program works best with the strength-training routines prescribed, *no aerobics added.* If you insist, however, you'll be doing less damage by performing your aerobic endeavor after your strength training on the same day.

CARDIOVASCULAR STRENGTH TRAINING

Please do not conclude from my discussion of aerobics that I consider the cardiovascular system unimportant. As I stated previously, it is very important. It is a critical part of human life.

But many aerobic experts would have you believe that the cardiovascular

---

DON'T MISTAKE RECREATION FOR EXERCISE

Many men impede their physiological progress by confusing exercise with recreation. They believe that raking leaves, having a picnic outing, or playing a few sets of tennis is an exercise endeavor. Any time they perspire, or their breathing becomes labored, they think they've exercised.

To get the most out of your Living-Longer-Stronger program, think of exercise as being a strategy enacted to bring about physiological improvement—that improvement being performing better, looking better, and feeling better. It must be an endeavor in which your body does demanding work in an anatomically correct manner to safely fatigue the muscles to an extent that stimulates growth.

The primary purpose of recreation is not to produce physiological improvement, but to provide fun. The exertion of playing tennis or other sports may produce some physiological benefit, but its occurrence is erratic.

If you're trying to get in shape by playing a sport, you'll probably suffer an injury before shedding the excess pounds you desire to lose and attaining an improved fitness level. As Dr. Fred Allman, a former president of the American College of Sports Medicine, notes: "You should get in shape to play sports, and not play sports to get in shape."

If you confuse and mix exercise and recreation, three undesirable consequences are likely:

- You will grossly compromise any forthcoming benefits of the exercise.
- You will destroy a large degree of the fun that recreation provides.
- You will make both more hazardous than they need to be.

The proper blend of exercise and recreation will be a bold step in the direction of Living Longer Stronger.

system comes first, if not exclusively. The need for muscular strength is placed well in the background. Even the aerobics people who practice proper strength training still insist on aerobics merely for aerobics' sake.

If you can see through the inconsistencies of aerobics, and at the same time experience the true effects of strength training, then a salient fact emerges. Proper strength training satisfies all the definitions of aerobics, with one exception. It does *not* provide the fun that is connected to the dance movements performed to popular music. And it never will.

Serious, productive exercise is not supposed to be fun.

If you strength train properly, you'll work your aerobic system efficiently at a high level, which will allow you to explore all kinds of fun afterwards. I promise!

8

THE IMPORTANCE OF A
MEDICAL EXAMINATION

In the front of all my fitness books, I include the following warning:

> The routines in this book are intended only for healthy men and women. People with health problems should not follow these routines without a physician's approval. Before beginning any exercise or dietary program, always consult with your doctor.

This advice protects both you and me. Obviously, we both want the program in this manual to produce the best possible results, while keeping the problems to a minimum. It may be in your best interest to get a health examination.

REASONS FOR A HEALTH EXAMINATION

There are four reasons you should consider having a periodic examination:

- *To detect unrecognized disease.* Every year, in the course of routine examinations, millions of persons are found to have previously unsuspected illnesses. The more important disorders detected and subsequently treated include diabetes mellitus, gout, silent heart disease, cancer, tuberculosis, and high blood pressure.

- *To evaluate physical fitness.* More and more medical examinations include various measures of fitness. To check your cardiovascular system, you are wired to a stationary bicycle or treadmill and asked to ride or run until exhausted. The thickness of your subcutaneous fat is calculated to determine your percentage of fat compared to lean body mass. Various tests are given that record strength and flexibility of certain body parts. These measurements are then evaluated according to norms for fit individuals of your age and occupation.

- *To establish a continuing doctor-patient relationship.* Even if no disease is found, your normal condition is recorded. As you age, things change. Appearance, weight, bodily functions, your electrocardiogram, your blood, and the results of other tests vary over the years. The observable differences between health and disease are sometimes very subtle. Certain minor variations in your electrocardiogram are usually of no significance. But if these variations are not present in previous tracings, they may indicate early trouble.

- *To provide reassurance.* To be reinforced in the feeling that you are healthy provides a peace of mind that cannot be measured in dollars.

WHAT THE EXAMINATION INVOLVES

What tests are performed and how reliable they are will depend upon where they are done as well as upon the experience and facilities of the doctor. At a large medical facility, a 40-year-old man requesting a complete evaluation would routinely have the following tests:

- Detailed history, which involves a written questionnaire

- Hearing and vision tests

- Chest X ray

- Rectum and prostate palpation

- Sigmoidoscopy, or examination of the lower bowel with an illuminated instrument

- Analysis of blood, urine, and stool

- Spirometry (breathing test) for smokers and asthmatics

- Resting electrocardiogram

- Stress-test electrocardiogram for overt or latent coronary heart disease

- Assessment of cardiovascular fitness from stress test

- Assessment of body fat, weight, and nutritional status

How Often

Opinions differ on how often you should have a complete medical examination. Some doctors believe examinations should be done on a regular basis. Others think there is no use to look for trouble as long as you are feeling well.

Complete examinations would be practical every three to five years after age 40, every two to three years after age 50, and annually after age 60.

If you are serious about the Living-Longer-Stronger program, and if you haven't had a complete medical examination within the last twelve months, schedule one today.

Play it safe. Do it now!

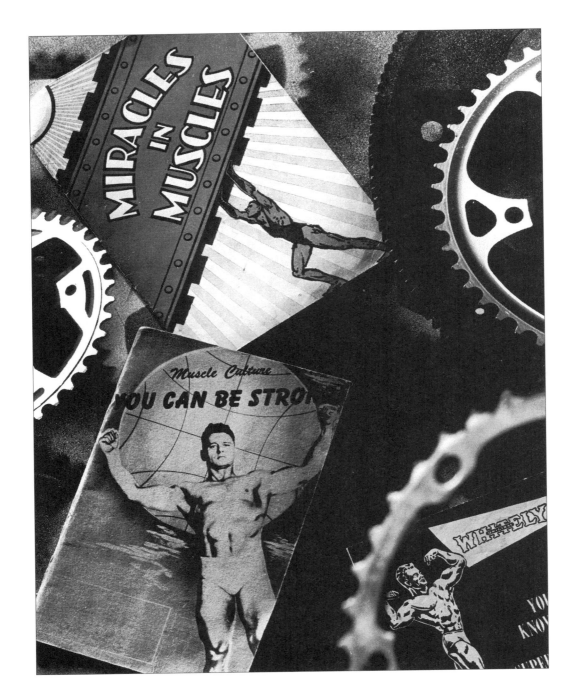

II.
REEXAMINING STRENGTH TRAINING

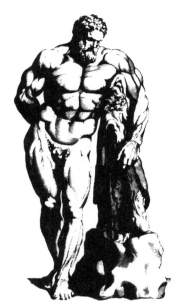

Hercules was a famous hero of early Greek and Roman mythology. This drawing by Hendrick Goltzius was inspired by a ten-foot marble statue called the Farnese Hercules, which is on display in Naples, Italy.

9

THE EVOLUTION OF
STRENGTH TRAINING

Men have probably always been interested in muscular size and strength. Why? Because we are mammals, and among males of most species, size is an indication of superiority. "Only the strongest shall survive" is a concept that certainly has prevailed throughout the history of mankind.

LOOKING BACK

The earliest records of formalized strength training can be traced to more than 4,500 years ago. Athletic contests often involved hand-to-hand combat and wrestling. Wrestlers were often depicted exercising with logs, rocks, bags, and even animals.

The major problem in early strength training was the nonprogressive nature of the tools. If a man was too weak to lift a certain log, he could not exercise with it. If he could lift the log, he could progress only in the manner in which he lifted it. Even if he had access to different-sized logs and rocks, systematic progression was crude at best.

Hand-held weights, similar today to what we call dumbbells, were utilized in Greek sports festivals in the sixth century B.C. This type of athletic exercise was practiced for hundreds of years, but was supplanted by the Romans with training that was more practical and dignified from a military standpoint.

References to weightlifting demonstrations can be traced to the late 1700s in German and British literature. In the United States, Benjamin Franklin in 1772 recommended dumbbell training because it contained "a great quantity of exercise in a handful of minutes." The dumbbells of that day, however, were rather light since they were made of wood or sand in bags. Iron dumbbells were scarce.

THE INFLUENCE OF GEORGE WINDSHIP

In 1865 George B. Windship, a medical doctor from Harvard, patented and offered for sale a plate-loading graduated dumbbell. The dumbbell could be adjusted in weight from 8 to 101 pounds. That same year Dr. Windship also sold an exercise machine, which he called the Health Lift. The Health Lift involved standing on a special three-foot high box or platform, which contained a small handle mounted on a vertical bar about two feet long in the middle of the box. The bar was connected to a weight stack underneath. By standing on the platform, straddling the bar, and grasping the handles, you could do a hip and thigh lift. Such lifting with several hundred pounds or more was considered by Windship to be very healthy for the human body. In 1866 in Boston, Dr. Windship opened America's first combination gymnasium and medical office.

Windship's major rival in heavy training was David P. Butler, also of Boston. By 1870 Butler was manufacturing several models of Health Lift machines, and had franchised his system, offering converts a chance to open gyms using his equipment. Like Windship, Butler centered his system on heavy, partial movements for the hips and thighs. By 1871, the Butler Health Lift Company had five different branches in New York City, three in Boston, one in Providence, Rhode Island, and one in San Francisco.

When Dr. Windship died in 1876 at age 42 after suffering a massive stroke, those opposed to his theories on heavy lifting were quick to blame his death on his training methods. As a result, Butler's studios gradually closed and his machines were relegated to scrap metal.

Both Windship and Butler had been influenced early in their lives by European strongmen who crisscrossed America as featured circus attractions. In many small towns, the circus was the only popular entertainment seen in an entire year. Circuses, which included strongmen shows, continued to be popular throughout the late 1800s. Frequently, these circus strongmen would demonstrate their strength by lifting huge barbells. These barbells, which they brought from Europe, consisted of long bars with large metal globes attached to the ends. These globes could be filled with various materials to make them heavier or lighter.

THE FIRST ADJUSTABLE BARBELL

Alan Calvert, a young Philadelphian and an admirer of the touring strongmen, wanted to get involved in weightlifting. Since no one in the United States manufactured barbells and dumbbells (Windship's and Butler's companies had gone out of business years before) and the European models were bulky, uneven, and dangerous, he started his own manufacturing concern in 1902, the Milo Barbell Company.

Calvert's weight sets included bars, sleeves, collars, and adjustable plates of 1¼, 2½, 5, 10, and 25 pounds. All of his equipment was sold by mail order, primarily through magazine advertisements.

The success of Calvert's company paved the way for the heyday of the mail-order, muscle-building era, from the 1920s to the 1950s, when men such as Charles Atlas, Bernarr Macfadden, George Jowett, Earl Liederman, Mark Berry, Bob Hoffman, Peary Rader, and Joe Weider popularized strength training through their products and writings.

In spite of the mail-order success of many muscle-building courses during the first half of the nineteenth century, most coaches and athletes in the United States were not advocates of strength training. Many coaches believed strength training would make an athlete slow and clumsy. Such a condition was often referred to as *muscle binding*, or *muscle bound*.

MUSCLE BOUND

The muscle-bound belief got its start from the touring professional strongmen. The average weight of these men was near 300 pounds at a height of less than 6 feet. Most of those who saw these men drew the erroneous conclusion that their ponderous size was a direct result of their weightlifting. They failed to realize that these men were for the most part genetic giants with hearty appetites. Another misconception was that since the lifting of maximum weights was usually done in a deliberate manner, the continued practice of such a feat would lead to habitual slowness in movement.

Furthermore, the year 1939 brought with it the first Mr. America contest, and subsequently other "muscleman" shows throughout the United States. Movie newsreels and newspapers often displayed the winners assuming tight, strained poses—which only reinforced the muscle-bound belief.

IMPORTANT RESEARCH

The muscle-bound belief was based on faulty assumptions. But from a scientific standpoint, there were no facts to disprove it. It wasn't until 1950 and 1951 that two studies, which were reported in the *Research Quarterly*, compared weightlifters against other athletes.

The first study concluded that a program of strength training increased athletic power to a greater extent than did a regular program of fitness activities. The second study revealed that weightlifters were faster in the arm movements tested than average people.

At the same time, Dr. Thomas DeLorme, an orthopedic surgeon for the Army Medical Corps, published several studies and a textbook: *Progressive Resistance Exercise*. DeLorme found no evidence that strength training produced a slowing of reaction time. Moreover, DeLorme's use of strength training for the rehabilitation of knee injuries during and after World War II began to get the attention of coaches, athletic trainers, physicians, and athletes throughout the country. Strength training was finally getting more positive attention.

GROWING POPULARITY

Throughout the 1960s, strength training became more popular. Most colleges and many high schools purchased barbells for their athletic teams. A multi-station machine consisting of several barbell-like exercises with self-contained weight stacks was introduced successfully by Universal Gym. YMCAs and fitness centers featuring weight equipment were opening in many large cities.

To meet this interest, several new bodybuilding magazines were published to blend with the regulars. Excitement was generated by writers who stressed routines involving words like blitzing, bombing, super-sets, double splits, iso-tension, burns, and retro-gravity reps.

Many times, however, the average trainee could not decipher what he should do from all the advice he was getting. Usually he did too much. In the end he didn't get the benefits he hoped for. Often he quit training altogether.

It was time for some sane, sensible, workable guidelines. It was time for Arthur Jones to emerge into strength training.

ARTHUR JONES'S CONCEPTS

I first heard of Arthur Jones in 1969. He had written a bodybuilding article that was published in *Iron Man*. That article was the most thought-provoking piece that I'd ever read in a muscle magazine.

Several months later, Jones self-published a revolutionary manual that he called *Bulletin No. 1*. I ordered this manual and quickly read it from cover to cover. Wow, I could hardly put it down. Within a week, I had read the book several more times and had underlined and starred concepts in almost every chapter.

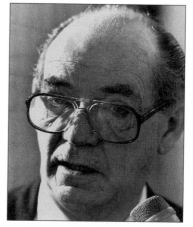

I met Arthur Jones in person in August 1970 at the Mr. USA contest in New Orleans. Within five minutes, Jones challenged my exercise beliefs and practices in a way that would eventually change my entire philosophy on training.

"The human body is exercised best," Arthur Jones said, "not by the volume of work but rather by the energy put momentarily into that work."

Then Jones hit me with five words: "Train harder, but train briefer."

Such a concept was difficult to comprehend, because during the 1960s athletes and coaches were bombarded with the more-is-better training. Nevertheless, I gave it a try under

Arthur Jones's harder-but-briefer theory started a trend in the 1970s that is still relevant today.

Jones's watchful eye. After just 20 minutes of pulling, pushing, stretching, contracting, and sweating, I could tell that Jones's style provided a superior workout. After a few months of his harder-but-briefer training, my physique was much stronger and leaner than it had been in the past.

NAUTILUS BEGINNINGS

In the meantime, Arthur Jones did more than expound upon a training philosophy. In 1971, he established Nautilus Sports/Medical Industries and began manufacturing Nautilus exercise machines. Nautilus machines were radically different from traditional exercise equipment. They were the first on the market to provide anatomically correct exercise.

In 1973, after finishing my work at Florida State University, I joined Arthur Jones as director of research and writing for his newly founded business in Lake

Helen, Florida. We planned, traveled, lectured, and worked on many projects together over the next dozen or so years.

By the mid-1980s, more than 9,000 fitness centers in the United States were using Nautilus equipment. More than any other single factor, in my opinion, Nautilus machines were responsible for the fitness boom between 1975 and 1985. Millions of men and women were turned on to strength training, most for the first time in their lives. (For a complete discussion of this phenomenon, see *The Nautilus Book*.)

In 1986, Jones sold Nautilus and started a new company called MedX. MedX manufactures clinical evaluation and rehabilitation equipment that primarily focuses on spinal pathology. Treating lower-back pain through strength training is Jones's current passion. MedX also sells a line of exercise equipment that is similar to Nautilus machines.

MACHINES OR BARBELLS?

It should be clearly understood that you don't have to have access to Nautilus, MedX, or any other type of machine to get significant results from the Living-Longer-Stronger plan. Barbells and dumbbells will work fine, if applied properly. If you do have machines available, however, use them. In fact, I'm going to show you how to use any type of exercise machine you have to your advantage, in a later chapter.

To get the maximum results from your strength training, you must remember Arthur Jones's harder-but-briefer discipline. In fact, I'll be reminding you of it throughout this book.

10

STRENGTH-TRAINING MYTHS

Old myths, even after science proves them wrong, often continue to thrive.

Such is the case with the muscle-bound myth, which I touched on in Chapter 9. A common belief still equates muscular development with being stiff, tight, and inflexible. It is true that some men with large muscles lack a normal degree of mobility. Large muscles can be developed through training regimens that do little to improve flexibility. In rare cases, the activity that made the muscles larger concurrently produced a loss of movement. But in the vast majority of cases, muscle size has a positive correlation to extensibility. When strength training is conducted properly, and especially when certain exercises and machines are used, the full-range movements that improve muscular size and strength simultaneously increase flexibility.

Besides the fear of becoming muscle-bound, there are many other myths that may discourage men in their second middle age from getting involved with strength training. Let's examine some of the most prevalent of these false beliefs.

MYTH: STRENGTH TRAINING WILL SLOW YOU DOWN.

If everything else is equal, the stronger, larger-muscled man will move faster because he will have a greater muscle-mass-to-body-weight ratio. Put a larger engine, with more horsepower, in an automobile and it will travel faster even though it weighs more.

Suppose you want to curl an 80-pound barbell as fast as possible. If your biceps muscle is capable of curling exactly 81 pounds, then your speed of movement with 80 pounds will be very slow. Perhaps five seconds will be needed to move from the extended to the flexed position. On the other hand, if your biceps is capable of curling 100 pounds, you'll curl the 80-pound barbell in half a second or less. If your curling capacity is 110 pounds, your speed of movement will be even more rapid. Since skill is not significantly involved in curling a barbell, increases in speed must be accomplished by strengthening the involved muscles.

The same holds true with movements not related to strength training. Any type of muscle-powered movement is met by some kind of resistance: air, water, gravity, or friction. Given equal resistance, the stronger man will invariably be faster.

MYTH: STRENGTH TRAINING TAKES TOO MUCH TIME.

Contrary to popular belief, properly performed strength training takes only 20 minutes per workout. Performed three times per week, that's one hour of training time for every seven days, or 168 hours. Investing one hour per week in exercise yields the best returns attainable in such a small amount of time.

MYTH: IF SOMETHING HURTS DURING AN EXERCISE, STOP DOING IT.

There's productive pain during exercise, and there's destructive pain. The productive pain is a burning sensation in the muscle that usually occurs during the last repetition or two of an exercise. High-intensity exercise works a maximum percentage of the involved muscle's fibers, increasing demand for nutrient importation and waste exportation. This is accomplished by elevated blood volume to and from the muscle. The muscle swells and becomes engorged with intercellular fluid.

Engorgement of the involved muscles impinges on various nerves and creates the burning sensation. Within minutes after termination of the exercise, the pain and burning dissipates as the engorgement diminishes. Such burning in the muscle should not cause concern. It merely indicates a highly effective exercise.

On the other hand, if you ever feel a sharp pain in a joint, *stop the exercise immediately.* Sharp joint pain can indicate injury to the joint and/or connective tissues. If the condition does not improve or worsens, see your physician.

MYTH: WHATEVER MUSCLE YOU GAIN FROM STRENGTH TRAINING WILL TURN TO FAT ONCE YOU STOP EXERCISING.

Muscle is muscle, fat is fat, and there is no way to turn one into the other.

Muscle is 71 percent water, 22 percent proteins, and 7 percent lipids. Fat is 22 percent water, 6 percent proteins, and 72 percent lipids. Like apples and oranges, muscle and fat are genetically and chemically different.

But why is it people fall for this myth?

When you stop training, you seldom decrease your caloric intake. The result is a gradual decrease in the size and strength of your muscles and an increase in body fat stores. Since muscle and fat are so close to each other that they can intermingle, it appears that your muscles have turned to fat. Fortunately, muscle and fat levels don't change immediately when you stop exercising. You can work back to your previous level in a fraction of the time it took you to get there.

MYTH: STRENGTH TRAINING INCREASES YOUR RISK OF CORONARY ARTERY DISEASE.

Strength training can reduce certain risk factors for coronary artery disease. Dr. Linn Goldberg of the University of Oregon Health Sciences Center studied the effect of strength training on fat buildup in the blood vessels. His participants trained three times per week for sixteen weeks. Results included a significant lowering of low-density lipoproteins (the "bad" cholesterol) and a reduction in total cholesterol levels.

Other studies also indicate that strength training, especially when combined with low-calorie dieting, can significantly reduce triglycerides, increase high-density lipoproteins (the "good" cholesterol), and lower the important risk factor of total cholesterol divided by high-density lipoproteins.

MYTH: STRENGTH TRAINING IS DANGEROUS FOR PEOPLE WITH HIGH BLOOD PRESSURE.

Many earlier studies determined that isometric contractions elevated blood pressure to very high levels. Some people, including physicians, incorrectly assumed that weight training did the same. This is not the case.

Dr. Wayne Westcott, fitness advisor for the YMCA of the USA, studied the blood pressure responses of over 100 subjects as they completed an eleven-exercise Nautilus circuit. He noted a small increase in systolic blood pressure and a small decrease in diastolic blood pressure, a perfectly normal response to rigorous exercise. He concluded that sensible strength training does not have an adverse effect on blood pressure in healthy adults. Dr. Westcott warned, however, that maximum lifts, breath-holding, isometric contractions, and hand-gripping can produce excessive blood pressure responses. Such activities should be avoided.

Researchers at Johns Hopkins University found that strength training can be a valuable method of lowering high blood pressure. They concluded that appropriate strength training is a very safe—but often neglected—mode of exercise for heart patients.

MYTH: STRENGTH TRAINING WILL MAKE YOU LOOK LIKE ARNOLD SCHWARZENEGGER.

This is a double-edged myth. Many younger men involved with body-building desperately want to look like Arnold. They read his articles and books, adhere to his routines, and eat his recommended foods and supplements. On the

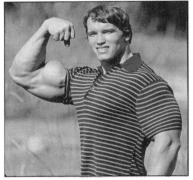

other hand, many older men do *not* want to look like Arnold. They find his muscularity unappealing, and they fear that strength training will overdevelop their muscles.

Both of these concepts are incorrect, and much of the reason centers around genetics. Genetics is an important factor in excelling in particular sports. For example, being tall improves your chance of being successful in professional basketball. For horse-racing jockeys, just the opposite is true. Your height can help or hurt you depending on the sport, but it's obvious that bouncing a basketball won't make you taller, nor will riding a horse make you shorter. Your height is primarily determined by genetics.

Arnold Schwarzenegger helped to popularize strength training by winning multiple Mr. Olympia titles, becoming an international movie star, and heading the President's (George Bush) Council on Physical Fitness and Sports.

Champion bodybuilders are born with the genetic potential to develop excessively large muscles. Muscular potential, like height, can be judged quickly if you know what to look for. The length of your muscles—from the tendon attachment at one end to the tendon attachment at the other—is the most important factor in determining their potential size. The longer your muscles, the greater the cross-sectional area, and thus the greater the volume your muscles can reach.

A long muscle presumes above-average size in that muscle. A short muscle implies that the muscle will be below average in size. Both extremes are rare. Having extremely long or short muscles exclusively throughout your entire body is seldom seen. Approximately one person in a million has such genes.

Arnold Schwarzenegger is one of those men. He has very long muscles throughout his entire body. Woody Allen, on the other hand, is an example of someone born with short muscles. Frame size is less important than muscle length in determining your ultimate muscular mass.

The majority of people have muscles that are neither long nor short, but average. Average-length muscles produce average-sized muscles, even after years of training.

If you have long muscles, you're probably already stronger than other men your age—even if you've never trained. With properly applied strength training, your results will be significant and rapid. Gains in muscular size and strength will be several times faster for you than for the average trainee, whose gains will always be more difficult to produce.

Don't worry about looking, or not looking, like Arnold. Recognize your genetic potential, then maximize it in the Living-Longer-Stronger plan.

THE FACTS ABOUT ANABOLIC STEROIDS

What they are: Anabolic steroids are synthetic variants of the strongest male hormone, testosterone. The most popular brand names are Decadurabolin, Sustanon 250, Primobolan, and Testosterone Cypionate. Nicknames include "roids" and "juice."

What they do: In conjunction with strength training, steroids stimulate the buildup of muscle tissue and improve recovery ability. They also increase aggression, which might make a person train harder.

How they're taken: Mainly in tablet form, may also be injected.

What they cost: Dosages vary widely. Users can spend $25–$500 a month.

How they're obtained: Legally, by prescription only; otherwise, several routes exist, including mail order. Mexico is a major black-market source, even though a large percentage of Mexican products are counterfeit. It is now a felony in the United States not only to use or possess steroids, without written medical clearance, but to encourage someone to do so.

How dangerous they are: When a person takes a hormone from the outside, the body becomes confused. It turns off its own hormone-producing system, so many peculiar effects occur.

    Brain: Increased hostility can lead to tranquilizer use, hypertension, and psychological dependence.

    Face: Facial hair growth and baldness in women; acne in men and women.

    Throat: Deepening of voice in women.

    Chest: Breast growth in men; breast cancer and decreased breast size in women.

    Heart: High blood pressure, high cholesterol levels, and clogging of arteries.

    Liver and prostate: Liver cancer in men and women; prostate cancer in men.

    Genitals: Sterility or atrophied testicles in men; menstrual irregularities, enlarged genitals in women.

The bottom line: While steroids may help your skeletal muscles grow faster, they are a time bomb ticking away at your heart, testicles, prostate, and other organs. Do *not* get involved with steroids.

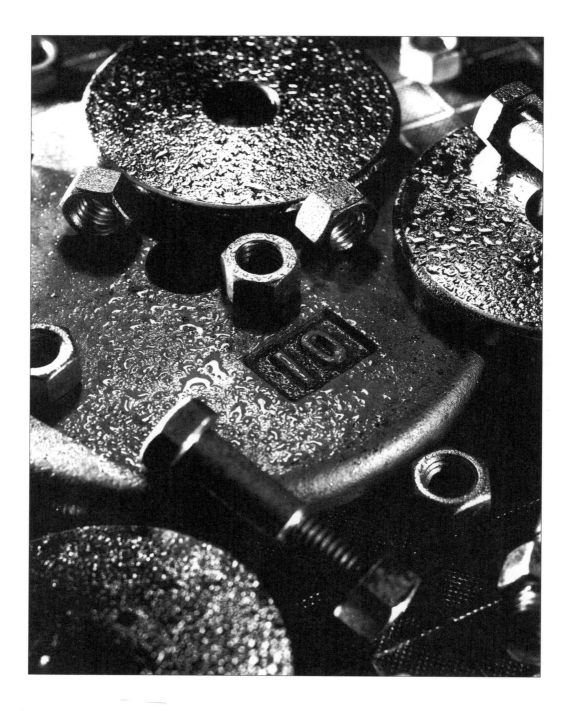

III.
REWORKING STRENGTH-TRAINING BASICS

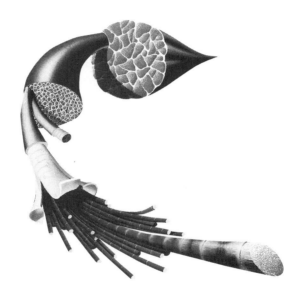

Bundles of muscle fibers (top) can be divided into myofibrils that can be subdivided into myofilaments (bottom). The myofilaments can then be separated into tiny protein units called actin and myosin, which have the ability to grow from proper strength training.

11
HOW MUSCLE GROWS

"You must first learn the basics." This is the command that every good teacher announces to any interested student.

Attaining proficiency in strength training involves the same process as in economics, mathematics, chemistry, and every other subject. You must begin with the basics. A clear understanding of the principles in Part III will assure maximum results from the exercises described in this book.

MUSCULAR GROWTH

Muscular growth can be best explained in a nontechnical manner by the use of two words: *inroad* and *overcompensation.*

Inroad is the depth of momentary muscular fatigue due to a strength-training exercise. For example, suppose you can do a one-repetition maximum in a barbell curl with exactly 100 pounds. Unload the barbell to 80 pounds and now perform as many repetitions as possible. Suppose with each repetition your muscles fatigue losing 2 percent of your original curling strength. As a result you can do 10 repetitions. At first the repetitions are easy because 100, 98, and 96 pounds of strength in your arms can effortlessly lift an 80-pound barbell. The last repetitions, however, are very intense and your attempt at number eleven fails because 80 pounds of strength won't lift a barbell of the same weight. Thus, you reduced your starting level of strength from 100 pounds to 80, or you made a 20-percent inroad.

Evidently some mechano-chemical threshold is crossed when muscle is inroaded to somewhere between 15 and 25 percent. Less than a 15-percent inroad doesn't work enough muscle fibers, and more than a 25-percent inroad may involve too many. There seems to be a fairly narrow balance between the minimum inroad required to effect stimulation and the maximum inroad the body can recover from. In any case, however, as a muscle weakens within these parameters it must momentarily fail in its attempt to lift the resistance. This combination inroad followed by intense failure seems to be the primary stimulus for the muscular growth process.

THE SCIENTIFIC SIDE OF MUSCULAR GROWTH

Your skeletal muscles are composed of millions of strands of a thin-filament protein called actin and a thick-filament protein called myosin. Given the presence of calcium, magnesium, and two other proteins called troponin and tropomyosin, actin and myosin can contract and move your limbs.

The fuel for muscular contraction is a chemical compound called adenosine triphosphate (ATP). When one of the three phosphates has broken off from ATP to form adenosine diphosphate (ADP), energy is released into the muscular environment. When actin binds to myosin in the presence of calcium, the energy released from ATP breakdown is used to pull the actin filaments along the myosin filaments. More specifically, a bridge forms between actin and myosin. Energy from ATP breakdown is used to shorten the actomyosin cross-bridge, which contracts the muscle.

There are a number of physical changes seen with hypertrophy that explain increased muscular size and strength:

- The actin and particularly the myosin protein filaments increase in size.

- The number of actin and myosin units increases.

- The number of blood capillaries within the fiber may increase.

- The amount of connective tissue may increase.

Before muscular growth is complete, overcompensation must occur. In other words, your inroaded strength not only recovers to your previous level of 100 pounds, but it must increase slightly beyond. Your fatigued muscle compensates back to 100 pounds, and then overcompensates to 101, 102, or even 103 pounds of strength.

Within seconds after you complete an exercise, your inroaded muscle starts recovering. Compensation usually requires a minimum of 24 hours. Overcompensation, especially if it involves multiple exercise inroads, normally takes 48 hours.

Your time between strength-training sessions obviously is a salient factor. The growth stimulation takes place during the exercise inroading. But the actual growing or overcompensation occurs after the exercise. Overcompensation requires time and rest.

THE IGNORED KEY TO MUSCULAR GROWTH

I learned the hard way. It took me several years, numerous injuries, and multiple hammerings by Arthur Jones—but at least I learned. Most coaches, athletes, and fitness-minded people never make the connection, they never see the key:

that any more exercise than the precise amount required for optimal results is not merely wasted effort, it is counterproductive.

Remember, compensation precedes overcompensation. Recovery always comes before growth.

Recovery and growth both require time to be completed. When training is carried on too long, or not enough time elapses between workouts to allow for full recovery, muscular growth will not occur.

The amount of training is always a negative factor in your recovery ability. Thus, you must constantly strive to keep your strength-training sessions brief, as brief as reasonably possible.

MUSCLE-FIBER TYPE

Although over a dozen different classifications of muscle fibers have been discovered within the human body, scientists generally group them into two types. These two types refer to fatigueability, or how slow or how fast a muscle tires.

The first type is called slow-twitch fiber, because it is slow to contract but has the ability to continue working for long periods. People who have a high percentage of slow-twitch fiber usually excel as long-distance cyclists, swimmers, and runners.

The second fiber type is called fast-twitch, which is best suited for short-term, powerful contractions. Individuals with a high percentage of fast-twitch fiber perform well as sprinters, throwers, and jumpers.

Individuals vary in the number of slow-twitch and fast-twitch muscle fibers throughout their bodies. Individuals with a large percentage of fast-twitch fibers have greater potential for increasing muscular size and strength than do individuals with a predominance of slow-twitch fibers. Most people seem to have approximately equal numbers of both slow- and fast-twitch muscle fibers throughout their body. A small number, however, have as high as 90 percent from one fiber type.

Whatever your ratio, it is determined genetically and cannot be altered. Specific training does not change slow-twitch fibers to fast-twitch fibers or vice versa. In fact, the only way to be sure of your fiber type is to undergo a series of muscle biopsies where a small sample of muscle is taken from various parts and analyzed. Muscle biopsies are not practical for most people.

12
INTENSITY AND PROGRESSION

"Look for ways to make your exercise harder, not easier," says Arthur Jones, "and you'll get better results." One way to make exercise harder is by applying intensity and progression.

INTENSITY

Your intensity of effort must be high on the last repetition of each strength-training exercise. According to the protocol that I'll describe in the next chapter, this should happen during the ninth through the twelfth repetition, or at most the thirteenth, assuming that the resistance has been accurately selected. The involved muscles by this time should be barely able to lift the resistance. When they are unable to do so, they have reached momentary muscular failure. Such high-intensity exercise requires the appropriate number of muscle fibers for optimum growth stimulation.

MOMENTARY MUSCULAR FAILURE

Momentary muscular failure occurs when you can no longer move the resistance upward despite your best efforts. In other words, it is temporarily impossible to achieve another repetition in correct form. This level of fatigue is what you're trying to accomplish at the end of each exercise.

Building your body is a deliberate, controlled procedure. Foremost in this procedure is your ability to grind out the last several repetitions, the repetitions that are the most painful. Learning to endure the pain is necessary for maximum results.

ONLY ONE SET

When a strength-training exercise is performed in a high-intensity manner, one set gives your targeted muscles optimum stimulation. Multiple sets of the same exercise are not desirable. If you feel like doing more than one set, you probably didn't do the set hard enough.

PROGRESSION

Having learned to spell *dog*, you cannot then improve your spelling by practicing d-o-g over and over again. You must systematically attempt and accomplish different and harder words.

The same thing is true when it comes to your existing level of muscular strength. You cannot increase your strength by the mere repetition of things that you can already do. For strength stimulation, you must constantly attempt the momentarily impossible.

The backbone of proper strength training is progression. Progression means trying to increase the work load each session.

Begin with a weight you can lift 8 times. Stay at that weight until you can perform 12 or more strict repetitions. On the following workout, increase the resistance by approximately 5 percent.

Make sure that you do not simply stop an exercise because you've completed a specific repetition number. Always try one more repetition even when it seems impossible. Try continually to increase your intensity.

This process is referred to as double progressive training, because first you add repetitions and then you add resistance. As simple as this concept is, it is often ignored by many advanced bodybuilders and professional athletes.

Over many years, I've observed thousands of such men training. Usually, they select a given amount of resistance on an exercise and then perform a certain number of repetitions—stopping well short of the point of failure. Then, they rest a while and do the same thing again and again.

No amount of such training will ever produce anything approaching the results that are possible from a small amount of truly progressive exercise.

13
FORM

There is one simple thing that will instantly improve anyone's muscle-building results—slow down!

Slow down the speed at which each repetition is lifted and lowered.

Specifically, if you do each repetition half as fast as you normally do, you will automatically get better results. If you reduce the speed by another 50 percent, the results will be even more dramatic.

WHEN FASTER ISN'T BETTER

In my opinion, at least 90 percent of the people who strength train perform their repetitions in a manner that could be described as fast, jerky, and explosive. For example, a guy doing a bench press in this form would take the bar at arms' length over his shoulders, drop it quickly to his chest, and ram it back to the straight-armed position. This entire down-and-up excursion takes approximately one second.

Research proves that a slow, smooth lifting and lowering form on each repetition is much more productive, as well as safer. Why, then, do most men still train in a fast, explosive style?

DEMONSTRATING OR BUILDING

Too many men confuse demonstrating strength with building strength. If you are trying to see how much you can lift one time, such as is done in a weightlifting contest, then it is to your advantage to shorten the range, move explosively, and cheat to the maximum degree allowable. Doing so involves principles of physics, such as momentum, power, and leverage.

A weightlifting contest is one thing; a strength-building workout is a different matter. In a strength-building workout you are trying to isolate a certain muscle or body part and work it intensely until momentary muscular failure occurs. Strict, slow, smooth movement isolates and intensifies the muscle involvement. Consequently, this makes the exercise harder and more productive.

POSITIVE / NEGATIVE

In most strength-training exercises, your involved muscles contract and uncontract. When a muscle contracts or shortens, scientists often describe the muscle as *concentric*. Conversely, when the muscle uncontracts or lengthens, they use the word *eccentric*. Because these words tend to look alike, a more popular distinction has evolved.

Concentric is referred to as *positive* and eccentric as *negative*. In other words, as a muscle shortens the contraction is called positive, or sometimes positive work. When a muscle uncontracts the lengthening is termed negative, or negative work.

In a biceps curl done with a barbell or a machine, you perform both positive and negative work during each repetition. Positive work is involved when your arms are bending and raising the weight. Negative work comes into play when your arms straighten and lower the weight.

Moving a weight up is positive; down is negative. This is true for all strength-training exercises that are recommended in this book.

Research has shown that there are levels of strength:

- Positive

- Holding

- Negative

Using a barbell for a strength test, let's assume that you can curl exactly 100 pounds in a maximum effort. Your *positive* strength, therefore, is 100 pounds. If you can curl 100 pounds, then we know from much research that you can hold 120 in the midrange position. Thus, your *holding* strength is 120 pounds. If you can curl 100 pounds and hold 120 pounds, tests indicate that you can successfully lower 140 in a slow, smooth manner. So your *negative* strength is said to be 140 pounds.

The above example reveals that you can hold 20 percent more resistance than you can lift. And you can lower 20 percent more than you can hold or 40 percent more than you can lift.

Form, therefore, has a paradoxical influence on your response to strength training. Fast movement is associated with a higher rate of performance improvement (demonstrating strength) but a lower rate of muscle gain (building strength). By training in a fast, momentum-assisted manner you can lift heavier weights. But because more momentum means less muscle tension, your performance increases will be much greater than your growth increases.

Fast movement brings surrounding muscle groups into action to initiate and assist the lifting. Slow movement facilitates muscle isolation and intensity.

Slow repetitions reduce your momentum, and, as a result, you lift less weight. But the targeted muscle groups are fully responsible for lifting and lowering the resistance. Thus, greater growth stimulation is produced.

EIGHT-SECOND REPETITIONS

How slow should you move on each repetition?

The rate advocated for *Living Longer Stronger* is 4 seconds on the lifting phase and 4 seconds on the lowering. That's 4 seconds up and 4 seconds down, or 8 seconds per repetition. There is a smooth turnaround at both the top and bottom of the movement. This form works well on all the recommended exercises.

THE IMPORTANCE OF SAFETY

All men in their second middle age, years 40 to 60, should be concerned that the exercise they do is safe. Fast, explosive strength training is dangerous. I've seen too many athletes injured, some permanently, from it. My own body suffers from the residual effects of it even after many years of not doing it.

Avoid seeing how much you can lift one time. Even two- or three-repetition sets can be dangerous. Remember, your goal is to build strength, not demonstrate it. Building strength can be done safely, with none of the problems associated with demonstrating strength.

Adhere to slow, smooth movement for 8 to 12 repetitions. You'll get the best results quickly and safely.

14

DURATION AND FREQUENCY

How long should each training session last?

The various parts of your body may be categorized as follows: hips, thighs, calves, shoulders, back, chest, upper arms, forearms, lower back, midsection, and neck. Eventually, each of these body parts should be exercised at least twice a week. The total number of exercises per workout should vary from six to twelve depending on your age, level of strength, and the equipment available. Ten exercises per workout is average.

Each exercise should be performed for one set of 8 to 12 repetitions, or from 64 to 96 seconds, with 80 seconds being the average time. No more than 60 seconds should elapse between exercises. Gradually, you'll want to shorten that lapse between exercises to 15 to 30 seconds.

30-MINUTE WORKOUTS

A typical workout, therefore, should require between 20 and 30 minutes. None of the workouts described in Part VI take more than 30 minutes to complete. In fact, once you learn how to do the exercises, a training session will be closer to 20 minutes in duration.

It's to your advantage to concentrate on making your strength-training exercise harder and briefer. As a result your body will recover more completely and get stronger faster.

THREE TIMES PER WEEK

Strength training every day is not advised because your muscles require approximately 48 hours recovery time between workouts. Remember, your body has to have time to both compensate and overcompensate from the inroads you've made. An every-other day, three-times-per-week training schedule proves nearly ideal. Most people prefer a Monday-Wednesday-Friday workout plan, which allows them a lot of free time over the weekend.

Many bodybuilders split their routines into lower body exercises on Monday-Wednesday-Friday, and upper body exercises on Tuesday-Thursday-Saturday. Thus, instead of strength training three days a week, they work out six days per week.

I've found that the body responds best by working and resting it as a unit, not by parts. You can't eat and sleep for your upper body without involving your lower body. You can't assimilate, circulate, recover, and overcompensate for one or the other as effectively and efficiently as you can when you treat your body as a whole.

An overall body routine that is repeated three times per week is best for building muscular size and strength.

15
OVERTRAINING

The average American man is a notorious workaholic. To get ahead in the business world, he is expected to arrive early at his office, stay late, and put in overtime on the weekends. It shouldn't be surprising, then, that he carries these work habits into his workouts.

TOO MUCH EXERCISE, TOO LITTLE REST

Overtraining is the result of too much exercise and too little rest and recuperation. It can actually cause a reduction in muscular size and strength.

The key is to find a balance between overtraining, in which your body is too taxed to respond to the stimulation of high-intensity exercise, and undertraining, in which the stimulation itself is insufficient and there is no call upon the body to adapt by growing stronger.

RECOVERY ABILITY

Recovery ability has to do with the range of chemical reactions that are necessary for your body to overcompensate and become stronger. As I described in Chapter 11, each exercise makes an approximate 20-percent inroad into the involved muscles' starting level of strength. These combined inroads must be replenished and increased before the next workout is begun. That's why *time* and *rest* are so important. You're much better off getting too much, rather than too little, rest. The primary reason is that recovery ability does not improve in proportion to your strength.

For example, the average untrained man has the potential to increase his strength by 300 percent before he reaches his full potential. But his potential for increasing his recovery ability is only 50 percent. So comparing 300 percent to 50 percent reveals that your potential recovery ability is disproportionately small compared to your muscular strength potential.

The stronger you become, the greater the demands you are able to make on your recovery ability. In order not to overwhelm your recovery ability and to prevent overtraining, you gradually reduce the number of exercises and the frequency of workouts. Chapter 41 shows you specifically how to do this.

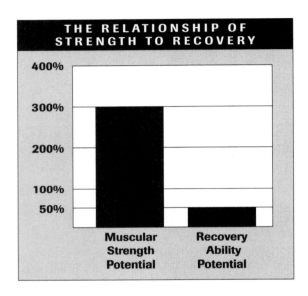

HARDER EXERCISE, LONGER REST

Most men assume that the stronger they get, the more exercise they need. But, in fact, when they reach a certain level of strength, they need shorter periods of harder exercise and longer periods of rest.

This prevents overtraining and maximizes your recovery ability.

And best of all, it builds larger and stronger muscles.

16
OTHER STRENGTH-TRAINING CONSIDERATIONS

Getting the most out of your strength training isn't the product of doing one thing 100 percent better. It comes from doing a lot of little things, each one 5 or 10 percent better.

This chapter deals with other little things you'll need to consider prior to starting a strength-training program.

APPROPRIATE STARTING WEIGHTS

Which starting weights will be appropriate for you to use will vary depending on your current strength, condition, and past experience. It's always best initially to select a moderately light weight—usually 20 to 30 pounds on a machine or simply the weight of the bar without plates—and concentrate on correct performance of the exercise. After one or two sessions of learning more than training, you can add resistance until you only do 8 repetitions in each movement. You'll now be ready to follow the double progressive system described in Chapter 12.

BREATHING DURING EXERCISE

Weightlifters frequently recommend that you inhale as the weight is lifted and exhale as the weight is lowered. Such a style may be helpful if you are demonstrating strength with a maximum lift. This technique, however, doesn't work well with the Living-Longer-Stronger form of training. Imagine with a slow, eight-second-repetition pattern trying to take one respiration per repetition for a minute or so. It simply doesn't work.

The correct way to breathe is to keep your mouth open, relax your face and neck, and breathe freely. Deep breaths are not necessary. In fact, it's to your advantage to practice shallow, rapid breaths with emphasis on blowing out rather than taking in large gulps of air. Try to ventilate just enough so your breathing doesn't stop.

Don't hold your breath during those last repetitions. Keeping your air passages closed while straining can elevate your blood pressure significantly and cause something called the Valsalva effect, which may lead to a blackout or headache.

Also, do not excessively grit your teeth, grip the equipment or grimace during exercise. These activities unnecessarily raise your blood pressure.

TRAINING PARTNER

Most men will make better progress in their strength training if they team up with a partner. In selecting a training partner, there are several things to keep in mind:

- Your partner should be similar in age and strength.

- Your partner should be *serious* about getting into shape and making a commitment to you. That commitment means you'll be exercising together one hour, three times per week. Each of your joint training sessions should take approximately 50 minutes: 25 minutes for your workout and 25 minutes spent supervising your partner's workout.

- Your partner should be someone with whom you'll share a spirit of cooperation, not competition.

- Your partner should not be your spouse, girlfriend, brother, or other family member. You do not want normal interpersonal problems to interfere with the training.

Once you have a candidate, it's important to explain how you want to be treated: strictly or loosely. Go over responsibilities and the roles you expect each other to fulfill. These include punctuality, weighing in, recording your workout on cards, reinforcing positive actions, and understanding and sharing problems.

While it's possible to make gains without a training partner, a motivated and serious person can make a great difference.

TRAINING RECORDS

Accurate records should be kept of your workout-by-workout progress. This can be accomplished on a card that lists the exercises with ample space to the right for recording the date, resistance, repetitions, and training time.

WHAT TO WEAR

What you wear to exercise in should reflect both function and your own personal style. Your workout clothing must be non-binding, allowing free movements of your arms and legs. Your clothes must also keep you warm when the weather is cold, and cool when the weather is warmer than usual.

One thing you should not go without in strength training is a sturdy pair of shoes, which are worn over absorbent socks. You should never train in bare feet or footwear without good arch support. The best workout shoes are called cross-trainers, which are widely available in athletic stores. Cross-trainers have both a solid arch support and good tread for gripping.

Many competitive bodybuilders these days wear leather or neoprene gloves to help with their grip during training. I've never liked wearing gloves, but I'm not against them if you're interested.

What I am against, however, is a leather or synthetic-fabric lifting belt. Wearing such a belt is not a good idea, especially if you are a beginner, because it keeps some of your midsection and lower back muscles from becoming involved in certain exercises. Rather than gradually strengthening weak midsection and lower back muscles, wearing a tight belt could actually weaken them.

WHEN TO TRAIN

There is no ideal time to train. Some men prefer to work out in the early morning, others in the late afternoon, and still others at night. It is best, however, to be consistent with your training time. Don't skip around. Get on a regular time schedule and stick to it.

Training can upset your stomach if you consume a meal too close to your workout. Allow at least two hours to pass between eating and training.

WARMING UP AND COOLING DOWN

I do not believe that an elaborate warm-up is desirable before a strength-training session. But I do recognize that the older you are, the more important the warm-up becomes. Smoothly performed calisthenic movements can be used as a general warm-up to precede your strength training. Suggested movements include the head rotation, arm circle, trunk twist, squat, and stationary cycling. Thirty to sixty seconds of each movement should be sufficient. In the Living-Longer-Stronger plan, specific warming up of each body part occurs during the first four repetitions, which take approximately 30 seconds, of each high-intensity exercise.

While some authorities recommend slow stretching movements as part of a warm-up, I disagree with them. Stretching should take place after the warm-up, not before or during. Or better yet, do it at the end of your strength-training session.

Cooling down after your workout prevents blood from pooling in your exercised muscles. After your final exercise, cool down by walking around the gym, getting a drink of water, and moving your arms in slow circles. Continue these easy movements for four or five minutes, or until your breathing has returned to normal.

17
FACTS ABOUT EQUIPMENT

Building the muscular size and strength of your body is dependent primarily on your understanding and application of intensity, progression, form, duration, and frequency. Another factor that can facilitate your results is your selection of strength-training equipment.

Naturally, I'm a little biased because for 20 years I helped develop and popularize Nautilus machines. But I've also trained with barbells, dumbbells, and many other machines such as MedX, Hammer, Cybex, BodyMaster, and Universal. Whatever the equipment, it's important to understand the mechanics behind proper exercise and correct machine design.

MACHINE DESIGN

Proper exercise of the human body requires movement against quality resistance. The highest-quality resistance has certain requirements:

- *Rotary*—Muscular contraction occurs in a straight line, and straight-line force is produced. But the body part that is moved by muscular contraction does not move in a straight line. Instead, the body part rotates, as it must, since it is working around the axis of a joint.

  For example, your biceps muscle on the front of your upper arm crosses your elbow joint. As your biceps contracts, it pulls your forearm and hand forward and up in a semicircular or rotary fashion. From joint extension to joint flexion, your biceps can rotate your forearm in excess of 140 degrees.

  Thus, a properly designed exercise machine for the biceps must provide rotary resistance. To do this it must have a movement arm that connects to an axis which in turn can line up with your elbow joint. In other words, the machine simulates the movement of your lower arm, and the resistance is always 180 degrees out of phase with the direction of movement. If your hand is moving straight up, then the resistance is straight down; if your hand is moving toward the east, then the resistance is exerting force toward the west.

In using any machine that provides rotary resistance, it is important to align your involved joint or joints in a coaxial relationship with the pivot points of the movement arms.

- *Direct*—Direct refers to the point of application of the resistance. Many exercise machines impose the resistance against several muscles simultaneously, which would be an advantage if all the involved muscles were of equal strength. Such is not the case, because the weaker muscles always tire before the stronger muscles are fatigued.

For example, in working the latissimus dorsi muscles of the upper back, it is necessary to bypass the weaker muscles of the hands and forearms. Gripping a bar or a movement arm, therefore, is a step in the wrong direction. What's required is to direct the resistance against the upper arms at the elbows. Thus, when momentary muscular failure is reached in such an exercise, it will be because the latissimus dorsi muscles are fatigued—not because the hands and arms are too weak to continue.

Direct resistance exercise machines place the movement arms against prime body parts, rather than filtering the resistance through weaker body part structures such as the hands and feet.

- *Variable*—Muscles are not equally strong in all positions, and movement produces changes in the mechanical efficiency of the joints involved. As a result of these two factors, you're much stronger in some positions than in others. If the resistance remains constant in all positions, it will be correct in only one position and too light in all other positions throughout a full range of possible movement.

A properly designed exercise machine not only supplies variable resistance, but it must vary in accordance with your potential strength in different positions. Most machine manufacturers provide variation in resistance by the use of a cam. A cam is a pulley with an off-center axis. It varies the resistance by giving you a mechanical advantage or disadvantage. So obviously, the exact size and shape of the cam is crucial. In fact, this one factor can determine the success or failure of some exercise machines.

Once you've become accustomed to a variable-resistance exercise machine, it should feel smooth throughout the full range of motion. If it doesn't, the cam on the machine is probably not correct.

In only a very few exercises do barbells and dumbbells offer rotary, direct, and variable resistance. Basically, barbells and dumbbells are unidirectional, allowing only straight up-and-down movement against resistance. This works in some exercises, but not so well in others. A properly designed machine, on the other hand, can guide your body into a series of twists and turns as well as ups and downs against rotary, direct, and variable resistance.

A machine can also supply your body with supportive structure, which can make many exercises safer to perform. Built-in weight stacks add safety and ease of adjusting the resistance.

Today there are dozens of companies that sell heavy-duty strength-training machines. Fitness centers, athletic clubs, and gyms are their primary market. If you have an exercise membership at one of these facilities, you have probably used some of these large machines.

RATING THE MACHINES

What's my opinion on all these machines?

I'm going to eliminate hydraulic and compressed-air-type machines because I like the visual feedback of seeing a weight stack being moved, which you don't get on these machines. Also, I'm not going to discuss the computerized exercise machines because, besides being very expensive, they are still not prevalent in most workout facilities.

Here's my brief evaluation, in the table below, of the most popular strength-training machines.

			Company Name				
		Nautilus	**Universal**	**Cybex**	**BodyMaster**	**MedX**	**Hammer**
	Rotary	A	A	A	A	A	A
Resistance	**Direct**	A	C	B	B	A	A
	Variable	A	C	C	C	A	B

STRENGTH-TRAINING MACHINE RATINGS

Note: All of the companies manufacture both rotary (single-joint) machines and linear (multiple-joint) machines. The ratings in this chart apply to rotary or single-joint machines.

A = excellent, B = good, and C = average.

From the ratings, you can see that all of the companies do an excellent job on the application of rotary resistance. On direct and variable resistance, only Nautilus and MedX get excellent ratings. The others score good or average.

Whatever type of machines you have available to you, you can still get results. How you use the equipment is much more important than the equipment you use.

18

THE BEST STRENGTH-TRAINING
EXERCISES

In my more than 30 years of strength training, I've probably tried every known exercise.

I figure, conservatively, that there are 400 different exercises or variations that you can do with barbells, dumbbells, and free-weight accessories (benches, racks, and pulleys). Add that to another 100 exercises you can do on the most popular machines, and the total is 500.

The exercises that best match the muscles' major functions become your basic strength-training exercises. In a nutshell, that's what I've done. From the possible 500 exercises, I've eliminated the overlapping, peripheral, and risky exercises, narrowing the list to 30 that really work.

The rest of this chapter is a listing of the 30 exercises according to body part. In Chapters 36 and 41 are detailed descriptions of how to do each recommended exercise in the most effective manner.

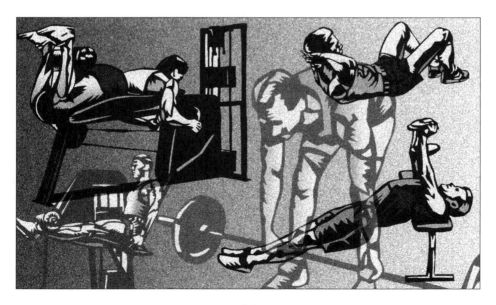

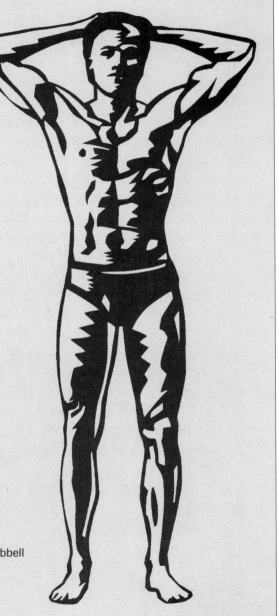

LIVING–LONGER–STRONGER EXERCISES

Forearms

Wrist Curl with Barbell

Upper Arms

Biceps Curl Machine

Biceps Curl with Barbell

Negative Chin-up

Triceps Extension Machine

Triceps Extension with One Dumbbell

Negative Dip

Chest

10° Chest Machine

Bench Press Machine

Bench Press with Barbell

Midsection

Abdominal Machine

Trunk Curl

Rotary Torso Machine

Calves

Standing Calf Raise Machine

One-Legged Calf Raise with Dumbbell

LIVING–LONGER–STRONGER EXERCISES

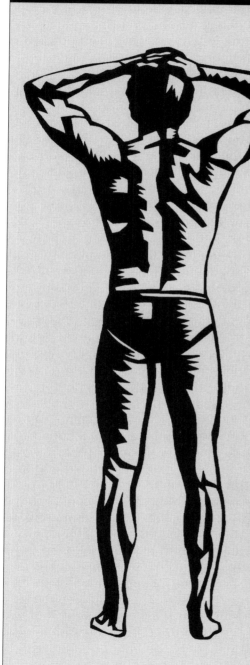

Neck

4-Way Neck Machine

Neck Extension Against
Hand Resistance

Shoulders

Lateral Raise Machine

Lateral Raise with Dumbbells

Overhead Press with Barbell

Back

Pullover Machine

Straight-Armed Pullover with One
Dumbbell

Behind Neck Pulldown Machine

Lower Back

Lower Back Machine

Prone Back Raise

Stiff-Legged Deadlift with Barbell

Thighs and Hips

Leg Extension Machine

Leg Curl Machine

Leg Press Machine

Squat with Barbell

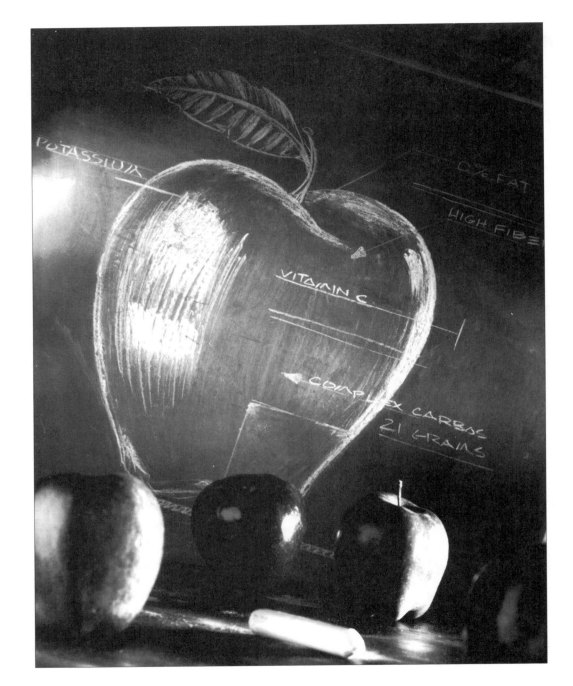

IV.
RELEARNING
FOOD
AND
NUTRITION

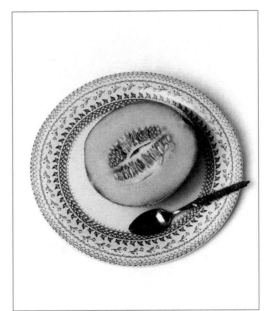

One-half of a cantaloupe contains approximately the same number of calories as an apple. But the cantaloupe is a richer source of essential vitamins and minerals.

19

PROACTIVE EATING

Proactive eating is a behavior that puts you in control of your food consumption. Such control is a result of not only your understanding of important variables, but actual manipulation of them.

The Living-Longer-Stronger program involves proactive eating. Applying this style begins with having a working knowledge of your nutrient needs.

RECOMMENDED DIETARY ALLOWANCE (RDA)

The RDAs are the levels of essential nutrients that are adequate to meet the known needs of all healthy individuals. These levels are established by the Committee on Dietary Allowances of the Food and Nutrition Board for the National Research Council.

These standards are revised every five to six years. Guidelines are listed according to sex, age, and weight for protein, eleven vitamins, and seven minerals.

It is important to understand that the RDAs are *recommended* daily averages. They are not requirements nor minimums, but they do take into account the differing needs of individuals. As a result, these allowances are several times higher than most people actually need. According to Dr. Fredrick Stare, founder of Harvard University's Nutrition Department, "intakes equivalent to half of the RDAs are usually adequate." Dr. Victor Herbert, a member of a past RDA committee, has noted that health hustlers often imply that individuals should consume more than the RDAs in case they have greater than average needs. Such is not the case because the RDAs are set higher to encompass individual variations.

FOOD-GROUP SYSTEMS

Remember the four basic food groups? Generally, this decades-old advice still makes a good foundation. The big difference in the system today is that the number of basic food groups is now six, and has been reconfigured as the Food

Guide Pyramid. A simplified version of the pyramid and information on recommended servings are as follows:

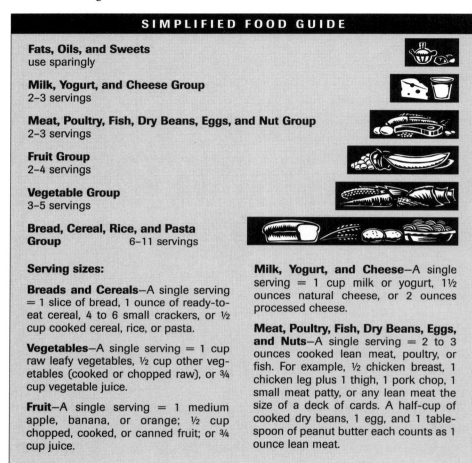

SIMPLIFIED FOOD GUIDE

Fats, Oils, and Sweets
use sparingly

Milk, Yogurt, and Cheese Group
2–3 servings

Meat, Poultry, Fish, Dry Beans, Eggs, and Nut Group
2–3 servings

Fruit Group
2–4 servings

Vegetable Group
3–5 servings

Bread, Cereal, Rice, and Pasta Group   6–11 servings

Serving sizes:

Breads and Cereals—A single serving = 1 slice of bread, 1 ounce of ready-to-eat cereal, 4 to 6 small crackers, or ½ cup cooked cereal, rice, or pasta.

Vegetables—A single serving = 1 cup raw leafy vegetables, ½ cup other vegetables (cooked or chopped raw), or ¾ cup vegetable juice.

Fruit—A single serving = 1 medium apple, banana, or orange; ½ cup chopped, cooked, or canned fruit; or ¾ cup juice.

Milk, Yogurt, and Cheese—A single serving = 1 cup milk or yogurt, 1½ ounces natural cheese, or 2 ounces processed cheese.

Meat, Poultry, Fish, Dry Beans, Eggs, and Nuts—A single serving = 2 to 3 ounces cooked lean meat, poultry, or fish. For example, ½ chicken breast, 1 chicken leg plus 1 thigh, 1 pork chop, 1 small meat patty, or any lean meat the size of a deck of cards. A half-cup of cooked dry beans, 1 egg, and 1 tablespoon of peanut butter each counts as 1 ounce lean meat.

This new food plan, introduced by the U.S. Department of Agriculture in 1991, designates fruits and vegetables as separate groups and recommends more servings of fruits, vegetables, and grains. Eating plans based on this system get most of their calories from carbohydrates and are limited in fats. You'll notice that the Simplified Food Guide provides more space to grains, fruits, and vegetables, than to meat and dairy groups.

At first, the number of recommended servings may seem like an enormous quantity of food. But a serving as defined by the guidelines may be much smaller than your usual helping.

The emphasis in proactive eating is clearly on carbohydrates. At least 60 percent of your calories each day should come from carbohydrate-rich foods. The remaining 35 to 40 percent of your calories come from proteins and fats, the meat and dairy groups.

Remember, the serving suggestions are meant as a guide rather than a prescription. Skipping one group entirely for a day or so shouldn't be harmful if your overall eating plan is on track.

GUIDELINES FOR HEALTHY EATING

From my study of the standard recommendations of the U.S. Department of Agriculture, the Surgeon General's Report, the American Heart Association, and the National Cancer Institute, plus my experience, here are my Living-Longer-Stronger guidelines for proactive eating:

- Keep your total fat intake at 20 percent of your daily calories. Limit your intake of fat by selecting lean meats, poultry without skin, fish, and low-fat dairy products. In addition, cut back on vegetable oils and butter—or foods made with these—as well as on mayonnaise, salad dressings, and fried foods.

- Limit your intake of saturated fat to less than 10 percent of your fat calories. A diet high in saturated fat contributes to high blood cholesterol levels. The richest sources of saturated fat are animal products and tropical vegetable oils, such as coconut or palm oil.

- Decrease your cholesterol intake to 300 milligrams or less per day. Cholesterol is found only in animal products, such as meats, poultry, dairy products, and egg yolks.

- Consume a diet high in complex carbohydrates. Carbohydrates should contribute 60 percent or more of your total daily calories. To help meet this requirement, eat five or more servings of a combination of vegetables and fruits, and six or more servings of whole grains or legumes daily. This will help you obtain the 20 to 30 grams of dietary fiber you need each day, as well as provide important vitamins and minerals.

- Maintain a moderate protein intake. Protein should make up about 20 percent of your total daily calories if you are trying to lose body fat. If you are trying to maintain your leanness, your protein can go down to 10 percent and your carbohydrates can move up to 70 percent. Choose low-fat sources of protein.

- Eat a variety of foods. Don't try to fill your nutrient requirements by consuming the same foods every day. Experiment with new and different foods—and read the labels carefully.

- Avoid too much sugar. Many foods that are high in sugar are also high in fat. Sugar also contributes to tooth decay.

- Lower your sodium intake to 2,400 milligrams per day. This is equal to the amount of sodium in a little more than a teaspoon of salt. Cut back on your use of the salt shaker and salt in cooking. Avoid salty foods; check food labels for the inclusion of ingredients containing sodium.

- Emphasize an adequate calcium intake. Calcium is essential for strong bones and teeth. Get your calcium from low-fat sources, such as skim milk and low-fat yogurt.

- Don't drink alcohol. Excess alcohol consumption can lead to a variety of health problems. And alcoholic beverages can add many calories to your diet without supplying other nutrients.

- Drink more water, especially if you are trying to lose fat. I recommend one gallon a day for most people.

Applying the tips to healthy eating is easier than you think. Here are some healthy meal recommendations.

BREAKFAST

Some of the best and worst foods in the American diet are consumed at breakfast. Such foods as bacon, sausage, butter, and cream cheese add considerable amounts of saturated fat to traditional breakfasts, while doughnuts, pastries, syrupy pancakes, and store-bought muffins add sugar, fat, and calories. Many cereals also provide hefty doses of sugar and sodium. And eggs, a staple of the American breakfast, supply one-third of all the cholesterol consumed in the United States. If your breakfast contains all the cholesterol or most of the sodium you should eat for the entire day, you may not be able to compensate for these excesses at bedtime.

It is probably easier to incorporate wholesome foods into your diet at breakfast than at other meals. Many low-fat, low-cholesterol foods are ideal morning fare, supplying nutrients that may be difficult to get in later meals. Breakfast is also an important source of fiber.

The foods that supply a good breakfast—and suit most Americans' eating patterns—are some form of complex carbohydrates, such as breads and cereals. Also recommended is fruit or fruit juice high in vitamin C, and low-fat or skim milk or other dairy products. A small amount of fat helps you feel full. Coffee or tea is harmless in moderate amounts.

If you prefer chicken and vegetables, that's great. What people eat for breakfast is largely a cultural matter. But you should try to get fruit juice, whole grains, and milk products at lunch or dinner if you leave them out at breakfast. Try to avoid foods high in sugar, which tend to be low in nutrients. Also, limit traditional breakfast foods that are high in fat, cholesterol, and sodium because of the damage they can do to your heart, arteries, and waistline.

LUNCH

For most men, lunch is a meal eaten hurriedly in the middle of a busy workday. As a result, you may tend to choose foods that are quickly prepared and convenient to eat: a sandwich and a bag of chips from the local deli, a slice of pizza, or a fast-food burger and fries. Many of these foods, however, are high in fat and sodium and low in fiber. Fortunately, you don't have to give up convenience for health. Most traditional lunch fare can be modified to be more healthful.

At home and at restaurants, sandwiches are a standard lunch. But some of the old favorites—ham and Swiss, egg salad, and pastrami—may be dealing out more calories, cholesterol, and fat than most of us want to consume at one sitting. To create sandwiches that are more nutritious, follow these suggestions:

- Whole-grain breads give you more minerals and fiber than white breads or buns. Most bagels and pita breads are low in fat as well as sodium.

- Processed sandwich meats such as bologna, salami, and liverwurst are usually high in saturated fat, cholesterol, and sodium. Roasting your own chicken or turkey for sandwiches is worth the effort. You'll cut down on calories, fat, and sodium. Discard all the visible fat on roast beef, ham, or pork.

- Instead of cheese or mayonnaise, add slices of vegetables or fruit.

- A tasty, low-fat sandwich dressing can be made with plain, low-fat yogurt, or by blending equal parts of low-fat cottage cheese and butter-milk, flavored with herbs and spices. A tablespoon of such a mixture has only 9 calories and a trace of fat.

- Catsup and prepared mustard are low-calorie, low-fat flavor boosters— 10 to 24 calories per tablespoon. But they are high in sodium, with 150 to 180 milligrams per tablespoon. You can make sodium-free mustard by mixing mustard powder with water. Prepared horseradish has half the calories and one-tenth the sodium of mustard or catsup.

Besides sandwiches, another lunch possibility is the salad bar. The salad bar is a nutritious addition to many delis and restaurants. Still, you must choose wisely, since most salad bars are stocked with numerous high-fat items.

To become a health-conscious salad-bar diner, keep the following proac-tive-eating guidelines in mind:

- Choose your selections carefully. For the most part, stick to vegetables, fruits, and legumes. Cottage cheese can also be a good choice, provided it is the low-fat variety.

- Be aware that such foods as avocados, olives, sunflower seeds, bacon bits, cheese, and diced ham are high in fat and sometimes sodium. Use them sparingly. Think of such foods as condiments rather than the main focus of your salad.

- Avoid high-calorie salad dressings, or limit the amount you use. A typi-cal small ladle at the salad bar holds about two tablespoons of dressing. Two ladles of Italian, French, or blue cheese dressing contain approxi-mately 300 calories, almost all of them from fat. Try using lemon juice, or vinegar mixed with a small amount of oil, or a low-calorie dressing instead.

- Pre-dressed selections such as pasta or three-bean salad, marinated veg-etables, and tuna salad are often doused with oil or mayonnaise. These items are also more likely to contain added sodium. Ask the manage-ment before you make a meal of any of them.

- Some salad bars offer hot foods as well. Many, such as macaroni and cheese, fried chicken, and meatballs, are high in fat and sodium.

However, roast chicken or turkey would make a healthful addition to your salad. Soup can be another low-fat option if it is vegetable-based, though it is likely to be high in sodium. Cream soups and those made with beef are often high in fat as well.

DINNER

For many men, dinner is the most important meal of the day. Research shows that Americans consume 42 to 45 percent of their total daily calories at their evening meal. The foods eaten at dinner contribute a significant amount of nutrients to the diet, but also a large proportion of the day's fat, cholesterol, and sodium.

It can be difficult to change eating habits at dinner because it is the meal most likely to be shared with others. One easy way to start is to make dinner a lighter meal. In fact, most nutritionists recommend that you spread your calories more evenly throughout the day. Creating a more healthy evening meal doesn't mean you have to make drastic changes in the foods that you normally would eat. Here are some suggestions:

- Nutritious starters include raw vegetables—such as carrots, peppers, celery, and broccoli—with a dip made from low-fat yogurt, a green salad with low-fat dressing, or a chicken-based soup.

- Brown rice instead of white adds potassium, phosphorus, and fiber to your meal.

- Other healthful side dishes include steamed vegetables, grains such as wheat, pilaf, baked potatoes topped with salsa or low-fat yogurt, and legumes flavored with herbs and spices.

- A steady diet of dinners centering around red meat can contribute more fat, cholesterol, and protein than is healthy. Fortunately, there are many alternatives, such as light-meat chicken or fish.

- Traditional desserts, such as cakes, pies, custards, and ice creams, are high in fat and should be consumed in moderation. Better choices are fresh fruit, frozen yogurt, ice milk, and sherbet.

20
NUTRITION FALLACIES AND FACTS

From 1959 through 1969 I was a food faddist. I took thousands and thousands of dollars worth of vitamin and mineral pills, protein tablets, and exotic powders such as desiccated liver, kelp, and brewer's yeast. At the same time I avoided white bread, carbonated drinks, and ice cream. I was convinced that this eating program would help me become a superior athlete.

Where did I acquire these beliefs? The majority came from physical fitness and health magazines. According to these publications, most recent champions had followed such a program. I never questioned these concepts until I entered graduate school at Florida State University. In fact, I kept trying to find new ways or more concentrated protein supplements to be certain that I was consuming more than 300 grams of protein per day—about four times as much as I actually needed.

MEETING HAROLD SCHENDEL

During my first postgraduate year, I attended a seminar at which Dr. Harold E. Schendel spoke on the role of nutrition in physical fitness. Dr. Schendel was professor of nutrition at Florida State and had spent four years in Africa and elsewhere directing research on problems of protein malnutrition. He had more than seventy published papers to his credit.

To say the least, Dr. Schendel disagreed with most of my nutritional concepts and did not believe my special eating habits were necessary, beneficial, or even safe. According to him, a fitness-minded person did *not* require large amounts of vitamins, proteins, or any special foods.

Over the next several months we had many friendly arguments concerning my practices and his scientific beliefs. Finally, he suggested that we collaborate on some research using me as a subject. Great, I thought. Finally, I'll be able to prove to Dr. Schendel and other scientists that athletes like me really require massive amounts of essential nutrients.

For two months, I kept precise records of my dietary intake, of my energy expenditure, and how I felt. All my urine was collected and analyzed by a graduate research team in nutrition science.

NUTRIENT OVERCONSUMPTION

The results of this study started me thinking in a different direction. According to the RDAs, my protein need at that time was 77 grams per day. To my surprise, whenever I consumed more than this amount, the excess was excreted. Worse than that, it was also determined that since I had been consuming massive doses for many years, I had forced my liver and kidneys to grow excessively large to handle the influx of these proteins. Overly large liver and kidneys can cause several medical complications.

Further experimentation made it clear that when I consumed more than the RDA of various vitamins and minerals, excess amounts of these substances were also excreted rather than being used by my body. Similar observations had been made by nutrition scientists since the 1930s, but it took a personal experience to undo the brainwashing I had undergone during my early years as an athlete. The knowledge I gained while earning my Ph.D. in exercise science, combined with more recently published nutritional experiments, proved to me why optimum nutrition for athletic performance requires no more than a balanced diet composed of foods that are readily available at grocery stores and supermarkets. The only people who benefit from expensive supplements are those who sell them.

DISCOVERING THE FACTS

When champion athletes attribute their outstanding speed, strength, or endurance to a food supplement, it's perfectly natural for other athletes—or those participating in serious fitness programs—to pay attention. If a magic food, pill, or dietary regimen might change you quickly into a world champion, why not give it a try? It may be natural, but it's still a mistake. I've interviewed athletes at three Olympic Games and I've trained many world-class amateurs and professionals, but I've yet to meet a single such man who had an understanding of what happens to his favorite foodstuff after it enters his body. Such athletes obtain their results in spite of their nutritional beliefs and not because of them.

I was successful for many years in bodybuilding, in spite of my nutritional practices. But I was even more successful after I realized that my consumption of excessive nutrients was totally unnecessary.

FOOD SUPPLEMENTS

A supplement is any food substance, or mixture of such substance, consumed in addition to or in place of food. The most commonly used food supplements are vitamin and mineral pills.

It is not legal to market any product with therapeutic claims until satisfactory evidence of its safety and effectiveness is presented to the Food and Drug Administration (FDA). Many nutritional products, however, are marketed as *dietary supplements* even though their intended use is for the prevention or treatment of a health problem. This intended use does not appear on the product label. It is communicated to retailers and customers through books, pamphlets, or word of mouth. Promoters of these products call them supplements, hoping they will be considered foods rather than drugs and therefore be exempt from the laws regulating the sale of drugs.

Promoters of nutrition fallacies and scams are skilled at arousing fears and false hopes. Four myths used to encourage the use of food supplements are as follows:

- It is difficult to get the nourishment you need from ordinary foods.

- Vitamin and mineral deficiencies are common.

- Virtually all diseases are caused by inadequate eating.

- Most diseases can be prevented or treated by nutritional means.

None of these concepts is true. It has been well established that eating according to the recommended guidelines is more than adequate for the health of the vast majority of adults.

VITAMIN AND MINERAL PILLS

People in the United States spend approximately $3 billion a year for vitamin and mineral supplements. Most people who use them believe they are getting nutrition insurance, but many also think that vitamins can provide extra energy, improve general health, and prevent disease. Those who take individual vitamins usually believe that these products have medicinal value in many areas.

Nutrition Insurance: Virtually all nutrition authorities agree that healthy individuals can get all the nutrients they need by eating a wide variety of foods. Most Americans believe this too, but at the same time many worry that their eating habits place them at risk for deficiency. This fear of *not getting enough* is promoted vigorously by food faddists and supplement companies. Too many people fail to understand that the RDAs are set high enough to encompass the needs of individuals with the highest requirements.

Perspectives on Food Processing: The supplement industry frequently promotes the idea that the processing of food removes much of the nutrients. This may be true to some degree, but usually the changes are not drastic. In fact, many processed foods are restored by replacement of destroyed nutrients. Furthermore, processing can make foods safer, cheaper, and often tastier.

Stress Vitamins: Some manufacturers have advertised that extra vitamins are needed to protect against physical or mental stress. Typically, stress vitamins contain ten times the RDA for vitamin C and several of the B group. Although vitamin needs may rise slightly in certain conditions, they seldom rise above the RDA. Even if they do, they can still be met by ordinary foods.

Natural Versus Synthetic Vitamins: Many companies claim that natural vitamins are superior to synthetic versions. And naturally, they charge more for what's natural. Scientists know that vitamins contain specific molecules, and that your body makes no distinction between vitamins made in nature and those made in the factories of chemical companies.

PROTEIN SUPPLEMENTS

For years, the biggest misconception among athletes was the belief that strength-training and muscle-building exercise requires massive protein intake. I wish I had understood the facts about protein and muscle-building before I spent thousands of dollars on various food products.

There is absolutely no muscle-building, performance, or health benefit from high-protein supplements. You can meet your protein needs by eating several small servings each day of meat and dairy products. The RDA for protein, .36 grams per pound of body weight, is an excellent guide for adult men to follow. Thus, if you weigh 180 pounds, your protein need is 180 x .36, or 64.8 grams per day.

What about the highly advertised free-form amino acids? Won't they assist the muscle-building process?

Amino acids are the building blocks of proteins. There is no advantage, however, to taking free-form amino acids. Dr. James Kenney, a nutritionist at the Pritikin Longevity Center in Santa Monica, California, has noted that free-form amino acids are anything but free. For example, 100 grams of a popular amino acid powder retails for $26.98—which is $122.49 per pound. Similar amounts of free-form amino acids can be obtained from chicken breasts—which can be purchased at a supermarket for one-fiftieth of the price. When protein foods are consumed, your body breaks them down into their component amino acids and puts them to use where they are needed.

Regardless of what you read in fitness magazines, don't waste your money on expensive free-form amino acids or protein supplements.

HERBAL PRODUCTS

Americans spend more than $60 million a year for herb teas and various herbal products. Herb teas may be composed of a single ingredient or may be blends of as many as 20 different kinds of leaves, seeds, and flowers. *The Medical Letter*, a continuing-education journal for physicians interested in treatment methods, regards as potentially toxic the following substances: juniper berries, shave grass, horsetail, buckthorn bark, senna leaves, burdock root, catnip, ginseng, hydrangea, lobelia, jimsonweed, wormwood, nutmeg, chamomile, licorice root, devil's claw root, sassafras root bark, Indian tobacco, mistletoe, and pokeweed root.

While most herbs are consumed for their flavor, many are used for their supposed healing properties. These healing properties are usually described in pamphlets, magazines, and books. Practically all of the written material on the healing properties of herbs is based on hearsay and folklore.

Dr. Varro Tyler, professor of pharmacognosy at Purdue University, has researched herbs extensively in his book, *The New Honest Herbal*. He notes that as medical science developed in the twentieth century, it became apparent that most herbal remedies did not deserve good reputations, and most that did were replaced by synthetic compounds that were more effective. Many herbs contain hundreds or even thousands of chemicals that have not been completely cataloged. Some of these chemicals may turn out to be useful as therapeutic agents, but others could prove toxic. With safe and effective medicines available, Dr. Tyler concludes, treatment with herbs does not make sense.

APPROPRIATE USE OF FOOD SUPPLEMENTS

In general, food supplements are useful for people who are unable or unwilling to consume an adequate diet. For example, physicians often recommend various food supplements for the following persons:

- Very young children until they are eating solid food.

- Older children with poor eating habits.

- Children who do not drink fluoridated water—fluoride supplements are recommended.

- Pregnant teenagers, who are likely to need supplementary iron and folic acid.

- Pregnant women with a history of iron deficiency.

- Children who are vegetarians may need supplementation, especially vitamin B_{12}.

- Individuals adhering to prolonged, low-calorie diets.

- Individuals recovering from surgery or serious illnesses who have disrupted eating habits.

- Post-menopausal women who are prone to osteoporosis.

- Elderly individuals who lose interest in food and eating.

As you can see from the above listing, almost none of these descriptions apply to reasonably healthy men. There is one area of nutrition research, however, that is of particular importance to men in their second middle age: antioxidant vitamins.

ANTIOXIDANTS VERSUS FREE RADICALS

All the chemical reactions with oxygen that take place in your body's cells are essential to life. These oxidation reactions create as a by-product highly unstable molecules called free radicals. Although free radicals are generated naturally in your body, exposure to cigarette smoke and other environmental pollutants can also trigger oxidation and the release of free radicals. Reactions involving free radicals not only can damage your cell membranes, but they also have potentially cancer-causing and heart disease-causing properties. In other words, free radicals are bad news.

Good news, however, comes from the laboratory studies of nutritional researchers showing that antioxidant vitamins can block the action of free radicals before cell damage can take place. The primary antioxidant vitamins are vitamins C and E and beta-carotene, a form of vitamin A. Population studies and some small clinical trials reveal that groups eating foods high in these vitamins tend to have lower rates of cancer and heart disease.

Some researchers have suggested that the greatest benefit may come from taking in more antioxidant vitamins than the RDA specifies. Other researchers aren't convinced that the evidence warrants taking antioxidant pills as supplements.

The best advice is to make sure you consume fruits and vegetables daily that are rich in the antioxidant vitamins, such as sweet potatoes, carrots, spinach, broccoli, bell pepper, cantaloupe, and citrus fruits. If you decide to take an antioxidant supplement, make sure it contains no more than twice the RDA for vitamins A (beta-carotene), C, and E.

VEGETARIANISM

Over the last decade, men in the United States have significantly reduced their consumption of meat. In fact, the U.S. Department of Agriculture estimates that 10 million Americans now eliminate meat from their diets. People who restrict or eliminate foods of animal origin from their diets are called vegetarians.

The main reasons people choose the vegetarian alternative are because they believe it is healthier and more natural, they think it is more ecologically sound, because it takes less energy to produce vegetarian food than meat, and/or they practice religious or moral dictates that eliminate meat.

The vegetarian has the same nutrition task as any other person: to plan a diet that will deliver all the needed nutrients for a specific calorie level with plenty of variety. It is certainly possible to obtain all the nutrients required for vigorous health while adhering to a vegetarian diet. Careful attention, however, must be given to getting adequate supplies of protein, iron, and vitamin B$_{12}$.

Excellent summaries of the special problems of vegetarian eating are published by the Food and Nutrition Board and the American Dietetic Association. A good book on the subject is *The New Laurel's Kitchen* by Laurel Robertson and coauthors.

If you're a confirmed meat-eater, cutting down on meat could be a viable alternative to cutting it out altogether. This is especially true if you fill in the gaps with plant foods that are typically low in calories and saturated fat. The switch can be fairly simple—just eat one pork chop instead of two, or chili with beans instead of ground beef, or more pasta and tomato sauce and fewer super-sized burgers.

21

EXAMINING THE HEALTH OF HEALTH FOODS

Health foods are edible substances that are supposed to be particularly beneficial to your health. These products are sold in specifically named health-food stores, as well as many drug stores, department stores, and supermarkets.

To imply that good health is directly related to food is an oversimplification. Health is a result of many factors, just one of which is food.

Your body does not require any particular food. It uses some 50 nutrients in varying amounts. No nutrient is considered a health nutrient. But any nutrient that is required for human nutrition is essential to life and health, even though some are needed in very small amounts.

Let's briefly examine some of the claims and facts behind the most popular health foods.

CLAIMS AND FACTS

Alfalfa: Advocates of alfalfa claim that it contains certain nutrients that more common plant foods do not. Alfalfa actually has less nutritional value than most of the more popular vegetables such as broccoli, carrots, and spinach. Claims have also been made that alfalfa contains all of the essential amino acids, but this is untrue. Alfalfa tea contains saponins, which can adversely affect digestion.

Bee pollen: Bee pollen is supposed to be a perfect food, but it contains no nutrients that are not present in conventional foods. It is also touted as an aid to athletic performance, although actual tests on swimmers and runners have shown no benefit. Bee pollen can cause severe allergic reactions in susceptible people.

Bran: A fiber of wheat grain, bran is composed mainly of cellulose, an insoluble fiber. It is effective against constipation, but so are whole grains, fruits, and vegetables in the diet. The claim that wheat bran can lower cholesterol is false. Excessive intake of bran can cause gastrointestinal disturbances.

Chelated minerals: A chelated substance contains some ingredient that is chemically bonded to another ingredient. Minerals in chelated supplements usually are bonded to protein, which is claimed to enhance their absorption into the body. There is no scientific evidence, however, to support this claim. Individuals with a medically diagnosed need for mineral supplements can get adequate amounts from non-chelated forms, which are less expensive.

Choline: Not essential in the diets of humans, choline is a chemical compound found in many foods. Thus, even if you did require a dietary source, supplements would be unnecessary. Although research is being conducted concerning choline compounds in the treatment of certain brain disorders, use of supplements will not improve memory or counter the aging process, as claimed by faddists.

Coenzyme Q_{10}: Preliminary evidence suggests that coenzyme Q_{10}, a group of chemicals produced in your liver, may help keep atherosclerotic plaque from forming by acting as an antioxidant in blood lipid particles. But there is no evidence that coenzyme Q_{10} supplements prevent aging or even increase enzyme levels in body tissues.

Enzymes: Many products containing enzymes are marketed with claims that they can enhance body processes. Enzymes are proteins that act as catalysts in your body. Enzymes present in food are treated in your body the same way as any other protein: your body digests them into smaller constituents. Thus, enzymes taken orally cannot function the same as enzymes outside your digestive tract. Such enzymes do not enter your circulatory system intact. The tiny amounts of amino acids they provide make no significant nutritional contribution. Pancreatic enzymes have some legitimate medical uses in diseases that cause decreased secretion of pancreatic enzymes into your intestine, but these diseases are not appropriate for self-diagnosis or self-treatment.

Fish-oil capsules: Epidemiological research has found that Eskimos and others whose diet is rich in certain fatty acids have less heart disease than other Americans or Europeans. Other research has found that supplements of omega-3 fatty acids (found in fish oils) can help lower blood-cholesterol levels and inhibit clotting, which means they may be useful in preventing arteriosclerotic heart disease. However, it is not known what dosage is appropriate or whether long-range use is safe or effective for this purpose. Most authorities believe it is unwise to self-medicate with fish-oil capsules; they should be used only by individuals at high risk for heart disease who are under close medical supervision. Eating fish once or twice a week may be beneficial. The FDA has ordered manufacturers to stop making claims that fish-oil capsules are effective against various diseases.

Garlic: Raw garlic and garlic-oil capsules are claimed to purify the blood, reduce high blood pressure and prevent cancer, heart disease, and a variety of other ailments. Some studies have found that people given daily garlic and garlic extract had lowered their blood-cholesterol levels. The *Harvard Health Letter* cautions that any evidence of benefit is preliminary at best.

Ginseng: Ginseng herb is being promoted as a stimulant, aphrodisiac, and a cure-all for many diseases. There is no scientific evidence to support these claims. Some studies have found that many ginseng products contained little or no ginseng. The FDA requires that any product containing whole, ground, or powdered ginseng must be labeled for use only in tea.

Glandular extracts: These products, sold as food supplements, are claimed to cure diseases by augmenting glandular function in your body. Actually they contain no hormones and therefore can exert no physiological effect upon your body. If they did produce such an effect, they would not be suitable products for self-medication.

Honey: Honey is crude sugar, with only trace amounts of any micronutrients, but not enough to make it significantly more nutritious than sugar. Honey and table sugar are both made of fructose and glucose. Honey, being sticky, is more likely to contribute to tooth decay.

Inositol: This is a compound that is promoted as having vitamin-like properties. Inositol is not a B vitamin, and your body can manufacture all the inositol it needs. Contrary to popular claims, supplements of inositol will not alleviate baldness, reduce blood cholesterol levels, or aid weight loss.

Kelp: Kelp is a seaweed that is common in the Japanese diet. Tablets of kelp are prepared from dried seaweed and promoted in health-food stores as a weight-reduction aid, a rich source of iodine, an energy booster, and a natural cure for certain ailments, including goiter. Kelp is high in iodide, a mineral needed to prevent goiter. But iodized salt furnishes an adequate supply of this mineral to our diet at a fraction of the cost of kelp. Excess iodide can be detrimental to your health.

Lecithin: Lecithin is a chemical manufactured by your liver and is present in many foods, including soybeans, whole grains, and egg yolks. Claims that lecithin supplements can dissolve blood cholesterol, rid your bloodstream of undesirable fats, cure arthritis, improve brain power, and aid in weight reduction are unsupported by scientific evidence.

RNA/DNA supplements: In your body, RNA and DNA use genetic information to arrange amino acids so they'll make proteins and build tissues. Supplements of these genetic materials from animals are claimed to rejuvenate old cells, improve memory, and prevent skin wrinkling. When taken orally, they are inactivated by your digestive process. Even if they could be absorbed and reach the cells, they would not work because human cells utilize human nucleic acids, not those from lower animals.

Spirulina: This is a blue-green algae, some species of which have been used as a dietary staple in several parts of the world. Spirulina is similar to soybeans in nutrient content, and is now sold in capsules and tablets. It contains protein of fair quality plus some other nutrients, but nothing that cannot be obtained much less expensively from conventional foods. Despite claims by proponents, spirulina has no value as a diet aid or as a remedy for any disease. Courts have ordered several companies to stop making illegal therapeutic claims for spirulina products, but others continue to do so. Some products have been found to be contaminated with insect parts.

Wheat germ: This inner part of wheat is a good source of some nutrients: protein, several B vitamins, vitamin E, some minerals, and fiber. Wheat germ is neither a cure-all nor a dietary essential. It is amply provided in whole-wheat products. As a supplement, it is relatively high in calories and cost.

Yogurt: Yogurt is nutritionally equivalent to the milk from which it is made, but costs more. It is a good source of calcium, riboflavin, and other nutrients—as are all milk products—but it is certainly not a perfect food with magical anti-aging properties, as it is sometimes claimed.

THE BOTTOM LINE

Be alert to spurious suppositions concerning nutrient pills and health foods. Realize that many of the people who spread food misinformation are quite sincere in their beliefs, but also understand that where health is concerned, sincerity is not enough.

The products sold in health-food stores are not more nutritious than the standard products sold in supermarkets.

Have faith in food for what it is, not for what it is claimed to be. Eat nutritiously and moderately, and you'll have all the health that food can bring.

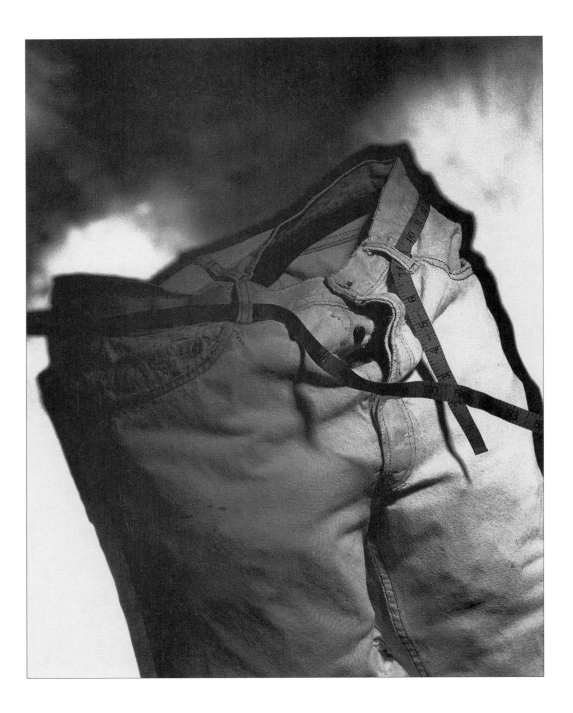

V.
REMOVING
EXCESSIVE
BODY
FAT

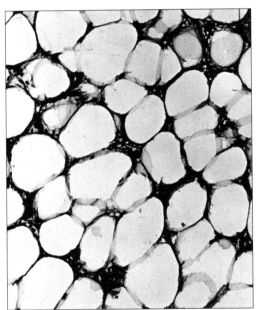

Viewed under a microscope, fat cells resemble a bubble bath. Each cell has the capacity to swell, when you get fatter, or shrink, when you become leaner.

22
MEN AND FAT

Not too many years ago, a man could lug his pot belly to a backyard pool party and actually show it off. Mass stood for power and durability, in cars and men alike. Remember those guys doing cannonballs off the diving board to demonstrate their bulk?

Times have changed, and for good reasons.

Besides being unattractive, a big gut is unhealthy. It can contribute to heart disease, liver and kidney problems, diabetes, and low-back pain. Plus, a protruding belly today makes climbing the corporate ladder more difficult. A lean waist in the business world denotes discipline, motivation, and patience.

PATTERNS OF FAT DISTRIBUTION

Men and women store fat differently. Men tend to deposit fat in the front of the body, particularly the abdominal region. Women tend to deposit fat in the back of the body, especially the buttocks and upper thighs.

Another genetic difference is that men tend to store more of their fat on the trunk rather than on the arms and legs, as women do. Much of the adipose tissue that a man accumulates on his front will be around the navel and over the sides of the waist. *Pot belly* and *love handles* are the familiar terms used to describe these conditions.

As almost everyone who has gone on a typical reducing program knows, you seem to lose weight from everywhere else first before it finally starts coming off your midsection. I know from my own attempts to lose fat that it comes off my love handles absolutely last. My normal body weight is 178 pounds, which includes the familiar love handles that I don't like. I can carefully work on a few things for about a month and get my weight down to 170 pounds. My waist will be two inches smaller, but those love handles are still there. Only when I get down to 168 pounds do those stubborn fatty deposits disappear. But I don't like how my face looks at 168, so I try to be satisfied at somewhere between 170 and 178 pounds.

It's a cruel trick of nature that we tend to lose fat last from the very places we'd like to lose fat the most. There's a reason for this, however, that is related to the fat cells themselves.

For a fat cell to be stimulated, it must have a receptor for the nerve action. Fat cells have two types of receptors, called alpha$_2$ and beta. The alpha$_2$ receptors increase fat storage, while the beta receptors stimulate the breakdown of stored fat.

Most men have fat cells in their abdominal areas that are rich in alpha$_2$ receptors. In other parts of their bodies, the fat cells are rich in beta receptors. This helps explain why belly fat is difficult to remove.

But don't give up just yet. With the Living-Longer-Stronger plan, I'm going to share many techniques that I've utilized over the years that will surprise you. Within your genetic potential, you'll be able to note some amazing changes in your waist and elsewhere.

ENERGY AND CALORIES

Energy is the internal power you must have for everything you do: breathing, sleeping, digesting, and exercising.

The sun is the ultimate source of energy. If you remember back to your high school physics, you learned that energy cannot be created or destroyed. It can only change its form and the place where it is available.

Plants have the ability to grow by combining the energy from the sun with the elements from the air, soil, and water. Animals usually get their energy from plants. Humans get energy from plants and animals. From a nutritional viewpoint, food and energy are measured in calories.

A calorie (kilocalorie is actually the scientific term) is the unit of measure for the amount of heat energy required to raise the temperature of one kilogram (a liter) of water by one degree centigrade. It is used to express the energy value of foods or the energy required by the body to perform a given task.

CALORIC VALUES OF FOODS		
1 gram of carbohydrate	=	4 calories
1 gram of fat	=	9 calories
1 gram of protein	=	4 calories

The energy values of foods are established by measuring the amount of heat given off when a food is burned inside specifically designed equipment. After years of experimentation, scientists found that the figures in the box were suitable for estimating the amount of energy supplied by various mixed diets.

The calorie expenditures for various types of activity have been calculated and written up in many diet and exercise books. It is well known that activity burns calories, and that if you are on a diet with a calorie limit that doesn't meet your body's energy demands, your body will find the calories it needs from your fat stores.

Losing fat, however, is more than a matter of simple addition and subtraction. It is true that any diet that contains fewer calories than you expend will cause you to lose weight. But unless that diet contains the correct balance of carbohydrates, fats, and proteins, much of the weight will not be from your fat stores. It will come from water supplies in your lean body mass—which is made up of your organs, blood, muscles, and bones. This is not where you want to lose weight.

Nutritionists have determined—and my research over the years has confirmed—that the ideal fat-loss eating plan should be balanced as follows: carbohydrates, 60 percent; fats, 20 percent; and proteins, 20 percent.

23

HOW FAT ARE YOU?

"He doesn't have an ounce of fat anywhere on his body."

Occasionally, you may hear this comment made about someone involved in fitness or sports, particularly a champion bodybuilder. But if you could do a careful dissection of his body, you'd find that he not only had ounces of fat, but pounds.

Fat is stored in many places throughout your body. About 50 percent of your fat is subcutaneous, which means that it lies in layers directly under your skin. Approximately 40 percent of your fat is marbled inside your muscles. The remaining 10 percent is around your essential and vital organs.

When a competitive bodybuilder gets very lean, he loses almost all of his subcutaneous fat. He still may have several ounces around his midsection and hips. His fat within his muscles reduces significantly, but he probably has a good two or three pounds remaining. His fat around his vital organs won't change much, which amounts to another two or three pounds. In his leanest condition, a 200-pound man would have at least five pounds of body fat.

So, even the most muscularly defined bodybuilder alive would still carry 2 to 3 percent of his body weight in fat. Even under extreme conditions of starvation, the body simply wouldn't allow the loss of its essential fat. Death would occur first.

MEASURING FAT

Statistics reveal that more than 50 million men in the United States are too fat for their best health and well-being. And most men gain 1.5 pounds of fat per year between the ages of 20 and 50.

How do you put a number on the amount of fat you have? Conventional height-weight charts are of little help, since they don't measure fat. Scientific methods that are meaningful include calculations based on X rays, potassium-40, ultrasound waves, underwater weighing, and electrical impedance. These procedures require special equipment and expertise and can be time-consuming and expensive.

The easiest, least expensive, and most popular method is to use a skin-fold caliper to measure the thickness of folds of skin and fat in various areas of your body. You can probably get a skin-fold assessment at your local YMCA, fitness center, or university exercise science department.

In the interim, you can get a fair estimate of your percent of body fat by using the pinch test.

THE PINCH TEST

1. Have a friend do the measuring if possible, because you cannot pinch your own skin-fold accurately.

2. Locate the first skin-fold site on the back of your right upper arm (triceps area) midway between the shoulder and elbow. Let the arm hang loosely at the side.

3. Grasp a vertical fold of skin between the thumb and first finger. Pull the skin and fat away from the arm. The fold should not include any muscle, just skin and fat. Practice pinching and pulling the skin until no muscle is included.

4. Using a ruler, measure the thickness of the skin-fold to the nearest quarter-inch by measuring the distance between the thumb and finger. Occasionally the top of the skin-fold is thicker than the distance between the thumb and finger. To avoid this, keep the top of the skin-fold level with the top of the thumb. Do not press the ruler against the skin-fold, because this will flatten it out and make it appear thicker than it really is.

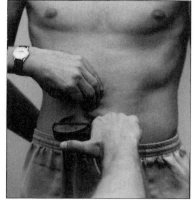

If you don't have access to calipers for skin-fold measurments, use a flat ruler. This photo shows the correct position for the second skin-fold site on the right side of the navel.

5. Take two separate measures of skin-fold thickness, releasing the skin between each measure. Add them together and divide by two to determine the average thickness.

6. Locate the second skin-fold site immediately to the right of the umbilicus, or navel.

7. Grasp a vertical fold of skin between the thumb and first finger and

follow the same technique as previously described.

8. Take two separate measures of abdominal skin-fold thickness. Add them together and divide by two to determine an average.

9. Add the average triceps skin-fold to the average abdominal skin-fold. This is your combined total.

10. Estimate your percent body fat from the chart below.

PERCENT BODY FAT	
¾ inch or less combined skin-fold thickness	5 - 9%
1 inch combined skin-fold thickness	9 - 13%
1¼ inch combined skin-fold thickness	13 - 18%
1¾ inch combined skin-fold thickness	18 - 22%
Over 1¾ inch combined skin-fold thickness	27 - 32%

Most men in their second middle age will be over 18 percent body fat. Many will have significantly more. Ideally, you should be 13 percent or less.

You can also take off all your clothes and look at yourself in a full-length mirror. Can you remember how you looked at age 20? How much did you weigh then? What was the circumference of your waist?

If you are typical, you were probably fairly lean and in decent shape when you started college. Your waist may have even measured 32 inches. Maybe those statistics from your 20-year-old body then can serve as useful goals now.

24
SPOT-REDUCTION DELUSION

Before going deeper into how to get rid of the fat, I'd like to clear up a lingering delusion about belly fat and love handles: *spot reduction.*

Spot reduction is a term associated with the idea that when you exercise a specific body part, such as your abdominals, the involved muscles use the surrounding fat for energy. This belief is the reason high-repetition sit-ups, side bends, leg raises, and twisting movements have been practiced for years as a way to remove fat from the waist. Unfortunately, such beliefs and practices are not based on scientific fact.

THE FACTS ABOUT SPOT REDUCTION

The fat that is stored around your waist is in a form known as lipids. To be used as energy, the lipids must first be converted to fatty acids. This is a very complex chemical procedure. To be used as fuel, the lipids travel through the bloodstream to your liver. In your liver they are converted to fatty acids, which are then transported to your working muscles.

It would be convenient if the fat cells selected were from areas where you have the thickest layers. But there are no direct pathways that exist from your fat cells to your muscle cells. When fat is used for energy, it is mobilized primarily through your liver from fat cells all over your body. The selection process your body uses for mobilizing its fat stores is genetically programmed. The mobilization process, in fact, operates in the reverse order from which you store fat. The last places you store fat are usually the first from which you lose it.

A typical man, for example, deposits fat first on the sides of his waist. It usually goes over the navel area second, then the hips, the back, and finally the thighs. When he starts losing fat, it comes off in reverse order—thighs, back, hips, navel area, and finally his sides.

Each person has a slightly different ordering of fat-storage spots. But that ordering is genetically determined and not subject to change.

Furthermore, I've already mentioned in Chapter 22 that men have more alpha$_2$ fat receptors in their abdominal region. Alpha$_2$ receptors facilitate the storage of fat, which makes the loss of it even harder.

SUPPORTIVE RESEARCH

Several scientific studies support the fact that spot reduction is *not* possible. One such study measured the skin-fold thicknesses of the arms of accomplished tennis players. If spot reduction were feasible, the more active—or playing—arms of the players would be significantly leaner than their inactive arms. Both arms of these tennis players were shown to be equal in fat content.

An even more convincing study compared the effect of abdominal training on fat-cell size. Abdominal, buttock, and upper back fat biopsies were taken from fifteen experimental and six control subjects before and after a 27-day abdominal exercise program.

Some subjects performed as many as five thousand sit-ups during this program. The results showed that fat-cell diameters decreased significantly at all three sampling sites, but there were no significant differences in the rate of change among the various areas.

WHAT MATTERS MOST

What really matters in losing fat efficiently is:

- The overall consumption of calories must be lower than the energy expenditure on a daily basis.

- The calories ingested should be correctly balanced from the major food groups.

- The calories consumed should descend gradually as the diet progresses.

- Combined with the three dietary facts above is the importance of muscle-building exercise to assure fat loss, increased metabolic rate, and improved body shape.

Even with the application of these steps, it is important to understand that fat losses come from throughout your body in disproportionate amounts according to your genetics.

SPOT REDUCTION, NO—SPOT PRODUCTION, YES!

While it is not possible for you to spot reduce fat cells around your waist, it is possible to spot-*produce* muscular size and strength in selective body parts.

Isolating and strengthening the right muscles can reduce flabbiness on your waist, give greater definition to your thighs and hips, broaden your shoulders, expand your chest, muscularize your upper arms, and improve your overall posture.

25
LOSING FAT THROUGH YOUR SKIN

What happens to fat when you lose it? How does it get out of your body?

I often pose these questions to groups of men who are interested in fat loss. Judging from the responses I get, most men are baffled, but intrigued, by the science behind the correct answers.

An understanding and application of the facts that follow will make all your fat-loss actions more productive.

LITTLE-UNDERSTOOD WAYS

Fat is energy, and energy is best expressed in calories. Remember, one pound of body fat contains 3,500 calories. Remember also from Chapter 7, when I made the point that no matter which energy system your body is using, it burns calories. Calories count significantly in losing fat.

Your body gets rid of fat or calories in three ways: through your skin, through your lungs, and through elimination of fluids as urine. Although you lose a small amount of heat through your feces, it is not thought to be significant unless you suffer from diarrhea.

Most of the calories are eliminated through your skin. Your skin is actually your body's largest organ, and as much as 85 percent of your daily energy emerges through it as heat. You lose heat through your skin by radiation, conduction, convection, and evaporation.

RADIATION

Heat radiates from the surface of your body. Whenever you are near something that is cooler than you are, heat leaves your body and is absorbed by that object. Or if the object is warmer, your body would absorb some of the object's radiant heat. Approximately 50 percent of the calories eliminated through your skin each day are as radiant heat.

A tall, lean person has a larger body surface area than another person who is the same weight but shorter and stockier. Because the tall person constantly loses more calories by radiation, he can consume more calories than the shorter person. Radiation is why shorter people tend to get heavier and taller people tend to remain lean.

Almost all of your skin's surface emits calories through radiation. The exceptions are where opposing surfaces of your skin limits exposure, such as under your arms. But nature has compensated by increasing the number of sweat glands in those areas.

CONDUCTION

Conduction of heat means the transfer of calories through direct contact. For example, when you get into a cold swimming pool, heat from your body immediately goes into the water. Water is a much better conductor than air, so you can lose more calories in cold water than in cold air. Conversely, if you are in a hot tub of water with the temperature higher than your skin, calories will be conducted to your skin's surface.

Various substances have different capabilities to conduct heat. Air, being a poor conductor, can be used as an insulator. Much of the insulation in new homes today works by trapping pockets of air between walls. Clothing is generally a poor conductor; thus, it usually insulates and keeps us warm. But we all have experienced the difference between wearing cotton and wool.

One tip concerning conduction that I learned years ago, from talking with Olympic wrestlers, is that shivering burns three times as many calories as sweating. Olympic wrestlers, before their final weigh-ins, are often frantic to lose that last half-pound of fat, which will guarantee a lighter weight classification. Shivering, they found, was the best way to accomplish this goal.

I've always encouraged my fat-loss group to adapt their bodies to being uncomfortably cool as they progress. This can be accomplished in a number of ways, even during sleep.

CONVECTION

Your skin disposes of another 15 percent of heat loss by convection. This means that air is circulating around your skin to move away the heat that has been formed by conduction. In other words, air movement helps with the elimination of heat. That's why the wind makes you feel cooler when you bicycle or walk. That's why an overhead fan in a workout room can benefit the cooling process as you exercise below. That's also why the wind-chill reading on a winter day is lower than the actual outside temperature.

EVAPORATION

Your skin perspires constantly, every second of every day and every night. Except when you openly sweat, you are probably not aware of this unnoticeable perspiration. The reason you are not aware is evaporation.

At ordinary room temperature, the moisture vaporized and lost from your skin, plus that from your lungs, accounts for approximately 25 percent of the calories lost by your body at rest. One-third of the heat lost by evaporation is removed through your lungs, and the other two-thirds from invisible perspiration on your skin.

Humidity, as anyone who lives in the South can testify, has a major effect on how efficient your skin is in transferring calories. As the humidity increases, your skin loses its ability to cool by evaporation. That's why sports and work in a combination of high heat and high humidity can be dangerous. When the humidity is high, your body has to depend primarily on radiation and convection to eliminate calories.

STRENGTH TRAINING CONNECTION

How efficient your skin is at eliminating calories depends on the blood flow through it. Your skin, as well as being your largest organ, is also very vascular. It is filled with arteries, capillaries, and veins. As you shrink your subcutaneous fat, the vessels in your skin will become more prominent.

The main purpose of this large vascular supply is to enable your skin to function as a means of controlling removal of calories, and thereby governing your body temperature. Here is where proper strength training comes into the picture.

There is no better way to condition your skin than to exercise the underlying muscles. With proper strength training, you can isolate and work any part of your body—from the little muscles of your feet and hands to the large muscles of your thighs and chest—which pumps blood to those specific areas. This surging blood brings nutrients and heat. The rising heat in the muscle must then be released through your skin. And your skin learns to adapt better by becoming a more efficient heat regulator.

TWO OTHER WAYS

Besides losing fat or heat energy through your skin, you also transfer it through your lungs and through your urine.

Approximately 10 percent of your daily calorie and heat loss goes through your lungs. Your lungs act as a bellows. Inhalation brings in oxygen-rich air, which is vital for energy metabolism. Exhalation carries out oxygen-poor air and the waste product, carbon dioxide.

The remaining 5 percent of your heat calories are lost through urine. In Chapter 27, I'm going to describe how you can significantly increase your urine production by drinking more water.

TRANSITION TO ENVIRONMENT

Let's briefly return to the initial questions and answer each specifically.

What happens to fat when you lose it? Since you can neither create nor destroy energy or fat, you can only transfer it. Thus, fat is transferred out of your body where it is put to use by other living organisms and by the environment.

How does it get out of your body? Fat is transferred from your body secondarily through your lungs and urine, but primarily through your skin.

Your skin deserves your respect!

26

SMALLER MEALS MORE OFTEN

If your goal was to get as fat as possible, in the most efficient manner, you'd be wise to eat one very large meal immediately before going to bed. In other words, you'd eat for only one hour out of every twenty-four. And that one hour would always precede sleep.

Sounds ridiculous, doesn't it? Who in their right mind would want to get as fat as possible?

FAT-FORMING EATING HABITS

In reality, many men in their second middle age have eating patterns that are not all that different from the above example. It's a pattern of: no time for breakfast, work through the lunch hour, eat a big dinner, and snack nonstop until bedtime. Millions of men starve their bodies when they most need calories and stuff them when they'll be doing nothing more strenuous than reading the newspaper and watching television. Such eating habits make no sense, unless you're trying to get as fat as possible.

BENEFITS OF SMALL MEALS

Research shows that losing fat in the most efficient manner requires just the opposite—eating smaller meals more often. Large meals of several thousand calories stimulate excessive insulin production, and insulin is your body's most powerful pro-fat hormone. Small meals bring on small insulin responses. Thus, it is advantageous to consume smaller-than-average-sized meals.

It makes little difference whether you consume four, five, or six small meals a day, as long as you are eating every three to five hours that you are awake.

It is more important to keep each of your meals to 600 calories or less. I've found that the calories above 600 seem to get stored more easily in most men's fat cells.

The meal pattern that I recommend during the first two weeks, the Living-Longer-Stronger eating plan, in Chapter 35, is illustrated below.

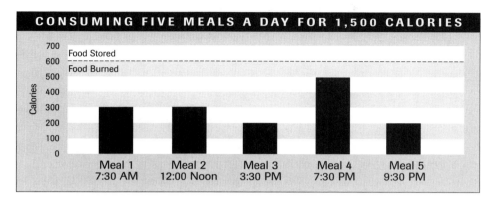

The Living-Longer-Stronger meal pattern involves a 300-calorie breakfast, a 300-calorie lunch, a 200-calorie afternoon snack, a 500-calorie dinner, and a 200-calorie late-night snack.

No Meal Over 600 Calories

Remember, eating smaller meals more often—with none of the meals exceeding 600 calories—is the best way to lose fat.

Keep your meals small, and your fat loss will be large.

27

WATERING YOUR FAT AWAY

Reading this chapter can make you thirsty. And it should. Water is your body's most precious nutrient. It's not only essential for life, but also necessary for efficient fat loss.

If you don't drink enough water, your body's reaction is to retain what water it does have. This, in turn, hampers kidney function, and waste products accumulate. Your liver is then called upon to help flush out the impurities. As a result, one of your liver's major functions—metabolizing stored body fat into usable energy—is minimized. Thus, a fat buildup occurs, water is retained, and your body weight increases.

To combat this fat buildup and to facilitate the loss of fat, you must drink more water than you probably believe you need.

MORE THAN EIGHT GLASSES

The standard recommendation for water is to drink eight 8-ounce glasses a day. During periods of fat loss and intense exercise, that's not nearly enough. That's why I recommend that men on the Living-Longer-Stronger program consume from 16 to 26 glasses (1 to 1⅝ gallons) of water a day. (The specifics of how to do this will be explained in Chapter 34.)

It may help you to purchase a plastic water bottle, the kind with a straw, readily available in supermarkets, service stations, and convenience stores. With such a bottle, you can carry water with you throughout the day for continuous drinking.

To further improve your fat-loss results, the water you drink should be ice cold. A gallon of cold water (40 degrees Fahrenheit) requires 123 calories of heat energy to warm it to core body temperature (98.6 degrees Fahrenheit). The water goes in cold and comes out warm.

Water is very important to an exercise program because it gives your muscles their natural ability to contract. From 70 to 75 percent of your muscle mass is composed of water. That's one reason you get thirsty when you exercise.

Water also helps to prevent the sagging skin that can accompany weight loss. Shrinking cells are buoyed by this fluid, which plumps the skin and leaves it clear, healthy, and resilient.

THIRST

You should drink plenty of water even if you're not thirsty. Responding to thirst will prevent only severe dehydration. It will not prompt you to drink the water you need to function at your peak.

Inadequate water intake causes the body to perceive a threat to survival, and thus it begins to hold onto every drop. Water is then stored outside the cells, showing up as swollen feet, legs or hands—what we commonly refer to as water retention.

The best way to overcome water retention is to give your body the water it needs. Only then will stored water be released.

If you have a persistent problem with water retention, even after drinking at least 16 glasses a day, excess sodium is probably to blame. The more sodium you ingest, the more water your system retains to dilute it.

One source of sodium not to be overlooked is your favorite diet soda. Although free from sugar, the sodium in diet drinks may cause water retention. Carefully check the labels to make certain these drinks contain little or no sodium.

FEELING FULL

Overeating can also be averted through water intake. Water can keep your stomach feeling full and satisfied between meals, thus preventing it from signaling your brain that you are hungry. When water is consumed in conjunction with foods high in fiber, this satisfied feeling increases because the fiber in these foods actually absorbs the water and swells in size.

CONSTIPATION CURE

Another desirable side effect of increased water intake is its effect on constipation. An article in a national magazine suggested that more than 50 percent of overweight men suffer from constipation.

Restricting your water intake makes you constipated. When deprived of water, your system pulls water from your lower intestines and bowel—thus creating hard, dry stools.

Water helps rid the body of waste, which is even more critical during periods of fat reduction since metabolized fat must be shed.

RUNNING TO THE BATHROOM

You're probably wondering: if you drink from 1 to 1⅝ gallons of water a day, won't you be running back and forth to the bathroom all day long?

Initially, for two weeks or so, your bladder will be hypersensitive to the increased amount of fluid. And yes, you will have to urinate frequently. Soon your bladder will calm down and you will urinate less frequently but in larger amounts.

WATER VERSUS OTHER BEVERAGES

There is a difference between water and other beverages that contain water. Biochemically, water is water. Obviously you can get it consuming such beverages as soft drinks, tea, coffee, beer, and fruit juices. While such drinks contain water, they also have substances that contradict some of the positive effects of the added water.

Soft drinks, coffee, and tea can contain caffeine, which stimulates the adrenal glands and acts as a diuretic. Some beverages are loaded with sugar and alcohol calories. In addition, too many flavored drinks can decrease your taste for water.

The way to interpret all of this is that your recommended daily water intake means just that—water!

WATER CONTENT OF TYPICAL FOODS	
Food	**Percentage of water**
Lettuce	96
Celery	94
Watermelon	93
Beer, regular	92
Beans, green snap	92
Broccoli	91
Milk, skim	90
Apples	85
Potatoes	80
Bananas	76
Eggs	75
Tuna, water packed	74
Macaroni, cooked	66
Beef steak, cooked	55
Hamburger, Big Mac	55
Cheese, Swiss	37
Bread, whole wheat	37
Bagels, plain	33
Butter	16
Crackers, soda	4
Cereal, oat bran	4

Tap Water or Bottled Water

In general, the United States has one of the safest water supplies in the world. Chances are high that your community's tap water is fine for drinking.

Furthermore, research shows that bottled water is not always higher-quality water than tap water. The decision to drink bottled water or not is usually one of taste.

If you dislike the taste of your tap water, then drink your favorite bottled water. If you have no problems with your city's water supply, then save some money and consume it.

A Final Note

Although it is doubtful that you could ever drink too much water (you'd throw it up or simply urinate more), a few ailments can be negatively affected by large amounts of fluid. Before consuming the recommended 1 to 1⅝ gallons of water a day on this program, play it safe and check with your physician.

28
WALKING AFTER YOUR EVENING MEAL

Walking, in my opinion, is not a productive activity for any component of fitness.

Walking does nothing for your strength or flexibility. It can produce a limited benefit on your cardiovascular endurance, but not efficiently.

Nor is walking an efficient way to burn calories. At least I didn't believe it was until I applied the results of a study by Dr. J. Mark Davis and colleagues from the Department of Exercise Sciences at the University of South Carolina.

Dr. Davis measured and compared the energy expenditure for three hours of seven subjects after the following treatments: exercise only, exercise-meal, and meal-exercise. The results showed that the meal-exercise routine increased energy expenditure among the participants by an average of 30 percent, compared with the other treatments. The researchers concluded that going for a walk after you eat brings on "exercise-induced post-prandial thermogenesis," which means the production of extra body heat created by exercising on a full stomach.

THERMOGENESIS—THE PRODUCTION OF HEAT

The study by Dr. Davis's group got me thinking about thermogenesis. I decided to review the scientific literature on the subject. To my surprise, several other researchers had studied the effect and found that taking a walk after a meal can speed up heat production by as much as 50 percent.

Had anyone studied the thermogenic effect of eating, exercising, and drinking ice cold water as a subject walked? I could locate no references. But the more I thought about it, I realized that combining all three had to be an even better way of producing heat and burning more calories.

THERMO-WALKING ROUTINE

After working with six groups at the Gainesville Health & Fitness Center, here's the thermo-walking routine that I found most effective:

- Eat your evening meal.

- Begin your walk within 15 minutes after you finish your meal.

- Walk at a leisurely pace for 30 minutes. How far should you walk at such a pace? A leisurely pace would cover from 1½ to 2 miles.

- Carry your insulated water bottle with you. Consume at least 16 ounces of cold water during the walk.

- Wear well-constructed, well-cushioned, and comfortable walking or running shoes. Do not wear street shoes.

- Dress in lightweight, comfortable clothes when you walk.

- Walk outdoors, if possible, on level ground. Or you may substitute a bicycle ride for the walk. If the weather is a problem, you may walk indoors, or use an exercycle or a treadmill.

WALKING FAT AWAY

Try the eating-walking-watering routine each day for the recommended six-week Living-Longer-Stronger plan and you'll be hooked on thermogenesis.

In a certain sense you'll be walking fat away!

29

THE IMPORTANCE OF EXTRA SLEEP

Most days, do you feel tired, draggy, or irritable?

If so, you're in the same bed with more than one-third of American adults. A recent Gallup Poll reported that one in three people are not getting enough sleep.

I need more sleep!

Millions of men make this complaint, but how many do anything about it? Sleep is a biological imperative, but do most men consider it as vital as food or drink?

Not in today's work-around-the-clock world. Not in a society where stores don't close, TV beckons all the time, and stock traders have to keep up on the action in Japan. For too many businessmen, sleep has become a luxury that can be sacrificed.

I challenge men in my six-week diet and exercise programs to get more sleep. Invariably the men who get the best results take me seriously, and accept my challenge. Extra sleep is necessary if you're dieting and exercising. Efficient fat loss and muscle-building both require a recovery time, and the best way to get the most out of your recovery time is to get more sleep.

UNDERSTANDING YOUR RECOVERY ABILITY

Recovery ability, as I noted in Chapter 15, is defined as the chemical reactions that are necessary for your body to overcompensate and get leaner and stronger. An optimum recovery ability is dependent on adequate rest, balanced nutrition, and sufficient time.

Your body is a complex factory, constantly making hundreds of delicate changes that transform food and oxygen into many chemicals needed by various parts of the system. But there is a limit to the chemical conversions that your recovery ability can make within a given time. If your requirements exceed the limit, your body will eventually be overworked to the point of collapse.

Years ago, sleep researchers focused on sleep as a brain phenomenon, ignoring the rest of the body. Now, they realize that sleep regulates the body temperature, replenishes the immune system, and yields hormones that facilitate fat loss and muscle building.

How much sleep is enough? Most men between the ages of 40 and 60 need eight hours. Only about 10 percent require significantly more or less sleep. Many of you, no doubt, are getting too little for your best performance. Most of you are certainly getting too little for the best possible fat loss and muscle-building.

SLEEP-REST FORMULA

Here's the formula concerning sleep and rest that has worked so well with men I've trained in the past:

- Go to bed an hour earlier each night, but get up at the same time as always each morning.

- Make sure your bedroom is dark, quiet, and comfortably cool. Studies show that sleep becomes more fragmented when the temperature goes above 75 degrees or falls below 68 degrees.

- Place your alarm clock so you can't hear it ticking in the middle of the night.

- Don't eat or drink anything with caffeine in it after lunch.

- Avoid alcohol. Although alcohol is initially calming, it interferes with the soundness of sleep.

- Take a 15-minute nap during the middle of the afternoon if possible.

- Shun vigorous activity on your non-strength-training days. Do not participate in tennis, golf, racquetball, or similar sports or fitness endeavors until you get your excess fat off.

REST MORE NOW!

Apply the guidelines in this chapter, and not only will you enhance your resting and sleeping, but you'll also significantly improve your fat loss and muscle-building.

30
OTHER FAT-LOSS FACTS

There are a lot of little things, none of which merits an entire chapter, that you can practice to speed up your loss of fat. Taken as a group, they can have a significant effect.

REDUCE YOUR SALT (SODIUM) INTAKE

The average man in his second middle age consumes many times more sodium or salt each day than required. The Food and Nutrition Board's National Research Council recommends 1,100 to 3,300 milligrams of sodium daily for adults. These levels are equivalent to ½ to 1½ teaspoons of table salt. With all the salt used in processed foods, cooking, and salting before eating, most men consume four to five times more than they need.

Aside from the relationships between excessive sodium and high blood pressure, and excessive sodium and fluid retention, salt generally hangs out with high-calorie foods. There seems to be an almost irresistible urge to eat foods that contain salt, fat, and sugar. And once you start, it's difficult to stop.

You can do your part by hiding your salt shaker. You won't need it for the duration of this program.

I'll do my part by providing you with an eating plan—which includes menus and recipes—that is low in salt. On the Living-Longer-Stronger diet, none of your daily menus contains more than 2,400 milligrams of sodium. This is plenty for even the most active man.

FILL UP ON FIBER

Although fiber is not a nutrient, it can be helpful in fat loss. Fiber, which is the tough, stringy part of plant cells, doesn't nourish your body because it isn't broken down fully during digestion. That's the key to its usefulness. Think of fiber as a broom. Its bulk helps *sweep* the intestine, aiding both digestion and elimination.

The recommended daily fiber intake for men is 35 to 50 grams per day. Most men usually get less than half the recommended amount. You'll get more fiber by emphasizing whole-wheat breads, whole-grain cereals, fruits, vegetables, and legumes. You'll learn how to consume more fiber in the Living-Longer-Stronger eating plan.

SLEEP COOL

Your body will burn significantly more calories each night if you sleep slightly cool. I'm convinced many men bury themselves under too many covers when they sleep. This prevents their normal thermostat from kicking in and supplying natural body heat.

If you tend to sleep with too many covers, try to eliminate one or two. Try to wean yourself from using an electric blanket and flannel sheets during the winter months, and during the summer, try only a single sheet on top of you. Soon you'll be burning several hundred more calories each night and forcing your thermostat to work harder.

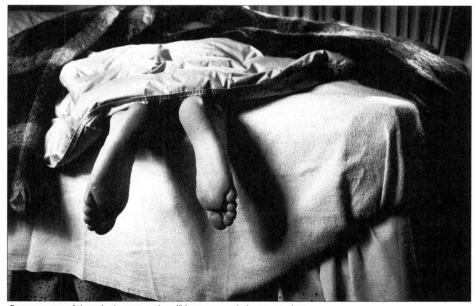

Remove some of those bed covers and you'll burn more calories as you sleep.

AVOID SAUNA, STEAM, AND WHIRLPOOL BATHS

Sauna, steam, and whirlpool baths heat the skin and cause profuse sweating, which can lead to dehydration. Dehydration does not contribute to fat loss or fitness. In fact, dehydration can actually cause your body to preserve fat.

Several times in this book, I've promoted keeping your body well hydrated and cool. Now, I'm advising you to stay clear of products that cause excessive sweating.

PRACTICE GOOD POSTURE

Forget the traditional *stomach in, shoulders back* admonition. Even the U.S. Military Academy at West Point abandoned this so-called brace position in 1968 after an Army study revealed it can cause a variety of problems.

The best posture resembles a marionette with a string attached to the top of the head. Imagine being tugged gently upward by the string. In other words, try to keep the top of your head on the ceiling. Automatically this straightens out the spine and tightens the abdominal muscles.

Practice sitting tall, standing tall, and walking tall.

BRUSH YOUR TEETH OFTEN

The next time you're really hungry, try brushing your teeth. It's much harder to eat with a clean, minty taste in your mouth. This is especially true if you crave something sweet and you brush with a tingly toothpaste. This tingly taste will cause anything sweet to taste bitter temporarily.

USE COLOR WISELY

Intense colors can stimulate your appetite. Don't use place settings or tablecloths of warm red, bright yellow, lime green, or orange. Even worse may be the red-and-white checkered tablecloths you often see in pizza parlors. You'll eat less on white or pastel plates and tablecloths.

CUT BACK ON YOUR EVENING TV

Watching television can hypnotize you to the point where you snack and don't realize how much you've eaten. Make it a personal rule never to eat while watching TV. Drinking water, getting outside for a walk, and going to bed an hour earlier will help you break the evening TV habit.

BEGIN A HOUSEHOLD PROJECT

To take your mind off food and keep your fingers busy, start a major project around the house. How about painting the garage, refinishing a table, or even washing and waxing your car? Any number of other undertakings would be just as good. Get involved and stay active.

BE ASSERTIVE

A leaner and stronger body automatically makes you more assertive. Practice saying *No!* when people offer you certain foods. Practice saying *Yes!* to things that are beneficial to your health. Soon you'll be in control—in *complete* control of your life.

31

AVOIDING OVERSTRESS

Mental or physical tension is called stress. A certain amount of stress is necessary for progress to occur. Too much stress, however, causes problems and breakdowns.

Most businessmen have experienced the stress that occurs in the corporate world. The popular press has circulated the fact that too much mental stress—especially extreme anxiety and grief—can trigger high blood pressure, depression, stroke, and even death. As a result, billions of dollars are spent each year in the name of stress by both researchers studying treatments and men seeking to be treated for the stress. Stress-management courses are now commonplace in many corporate environments.

The type of stress I'm referring to in this chapter, however, is the physical variety. Remember the example I used in Chapter 11 about making an inroad with each exercise? Making an inroad is a physical stress. The optimum inroad for each exercise is between 15 and 25 percent of your starting level of strength.

Less than a 15-percent inroad, and you have understress. More than 25 percent, and you have overstress. Obviously, your muscles thrive and grow from the proper inroad and stress.

Cutting back on your dietary calories is also a form of physical stress. And just as with strength training, there's a fairly narrow range of calories per day that produces the greatest fat loss. A moderate decrease of calories works much better than either a small or large reduction.

The importance of applying the correct amount of physical stress during a fat-loss program caught my attention during a Nautilus Certification Workshop held in New York City in July 1993. I have been on the faculty of these seminars for many years, and so has Dr. Wayne Westcott, a well-known researcher at the South Shore YMCA in Quincy, Massachusetts. Dr. Westcott and I both are interested in fat loss and muscle building. But, as a gifted runner, Dr. Westcott looks for ways to combine running, or aerobics, with strength training and dieting.

After listening to Dr. Westcott's presentation in New York, which contained his latest research on fat loss, I explored the idea of combining and comparing his data with mine.

COMBINING OUR DATA

What makes Dr. Westcott's and my data comparable is the fact that we've both applied the same eating plan with groups of subjects. The eating plan is from *The Nautilus Diet,* which contains a 1,250-calorie-a-day diet for women and 1,550-calorie-a-day diet for men.

Dr. Westcott studied groups of dieters who do aerobics, and groups of dieters who do aerobics and strength training. His groups who do the aerobics and strength training always lose more fat.

My fat-loss research included another group: dieters who do only strength training. No traditional aerobic exercise is allowed.

My data, published in *The Nautilus Diet,* followed 98 subjects (33 men and 65 women) through a ten-week diet and strength-training plan. For comparison purposes, the last two weeks were disregarded, since Dr. Westcott's groups were eight weeks in duration.

Let's examine the results:

COMPARISON OF FAT-LOSS RESEARCH		
Diet & Aerobics (Subjects: 22)	**Diet, Aerobics & Strength Training** (Subjects: 50)	**Diet & Strength Training** (Subjects: 98)
Fat Loss (Average in lbs.) 3.2	10.0	18.1
Muscle Gain (Average in lbs.) -0.3	2.0	2.4

As you can see, strength training plus aerobics provided three times the fat loss of aerobics only. Aerobics alone, in fact, produced a slight loss of muscle, which is not to anyone's advantage. Strength training alone supplied 81 percent better fat-loss results than a combination of strength training and aerobics; or 466 percent more effective results than aerobics alone. The strength-training group also had the greatest muscle gain in eight weeks.

Why is strength training combined with a reduced-calorie diet so much more effective for fat loss than dieting and aerobics, or dieting and aerobics plus strength training?

TOO MUCH STRESS

On a low-calorie diet, it is very easy for you to do too much exercise. Too much exercise is perceived by your body as overstress. Under such stress your body immediately starts holding onto fat. Fat provides security, protection, fuel, and safety. You must understand that much of your body's mechanisms are still being controlled by the blueprints that were established by your Ice-Age and more recent ancestors. In many respects, your body is survival-oriented.

When any of the following factors come into play, overstress is the result:

- *A very low-calorie diet:* under 1,200 calories a day for most men.

- *Too little dietary fat:* less than 30 grams per day for men.

- *Too much exercise:* longer than 45 minutes per day, or more frequently than three times per week.

- *Too little rest:* less than seven hours sleep per night.

- *Dehydration:* a loss of even 1 percent of the body's water can cause alarm.

- *Excessive heat:* high levels of environmental heat can reduce the body's efficiency.

- *Accumulated problems* from work or relationships that can also have negative effects.

- *Sicknesses, drugs, or extreme behaviors* that can send survival signals to the body.

STAY CLEAR OF EXTREMES

Instead of negative actions, you want to communicate to your body that everything is well. You do this by avoiding extremes and by practicing moderation, moderation in everything—except your exercise intensity. Moderately intense exercise is not very productive.

Your fat-loss exercise, as I discussed in Chapter 12, must be intense, as intense as reasonably possible. It must be brief in duration. High-intensity, brief exercise is responsible for muscular growth stimulation.

How does muscular growth stimulation send a positive message to your body to part with its fat? Once again, we have to return to our ancient ancestors for the answer.

MUSCLES AND SURVIVAL

One of the fundamental traits of our ancestors' lives was locomotion. Locomotion depended on muscular size and strength. Anthropological research shows that survival resources were allocated to the muscles first. An individual had to be able to run fast and fight fiercely to eat and avoid being eaten. In other words, hard, brief activity produced bigger muscles, and bigger muscles led to success at hunting and combat. Bigger muscles improved the probability of survival.

Today, when you go on an even moderately reduced-calorie diet, your body perceives that something is wrong. It kicks into its survival mechanism, which prevents you from losing fat in the most efficient manner.

To prevent this from occurring, you have to overrule your survival mechanisms by stimulating your muscles to grow with intensive exercise. Your growing muscles will then pull calories from your fat cells. Doing so significantly increases the effectiveness and efficiency of your ability to lose fat.

TAKE COMMAND

For maximum fat loss, take command of the salient factors involved. Practice strength training in a high-intensity fashion. Avoid having too much stress in your life.

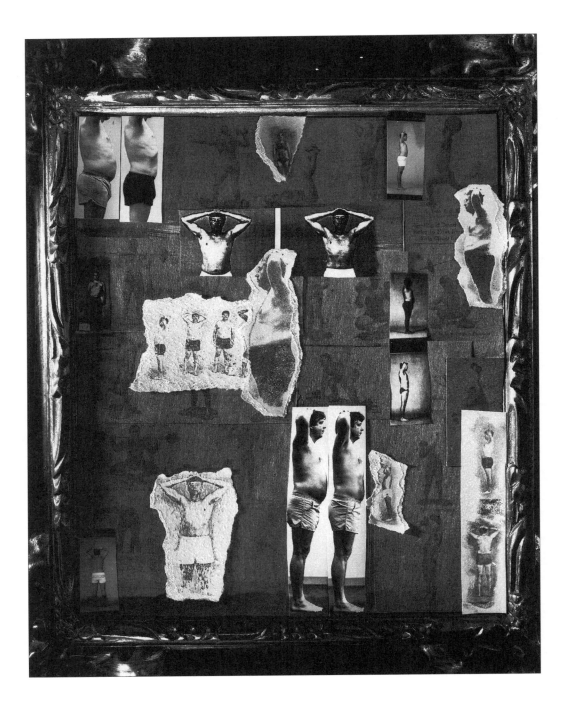

VI.
REBUILDING
AND
REDUCING
PROGRAMS

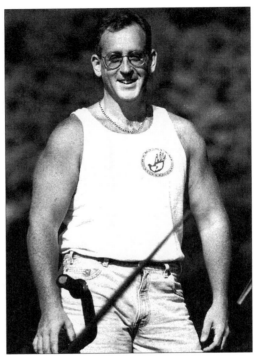

Larry Freedman accepted the Living-Longer-Stronger challenge. He applied the guidelines, mastered the discipline, and reaped the results.

32

52 Pounds and Counting:
One Man's Success

In March 1993, I confronted the members of the Alachua County (Florida) Sheriff's Office to get involved in my six-week diet and exercise plan at the Gainesville Health & Fitness Center.

Under my supervision, a small group was organized to meet every Monday, Wednesday, and Friday night at 8:30 p.m. The heaviest group member was Larry Freedman, who weighed 306 pounds with 45 percent body fat. Larry was 5 feet 11 inches tall, 29 years old, and had a waist measurement of 52 5/8 inches.

Larry loved sweets. And he liked to snack frequently at his sedentary desk job.

Larry and the others were placed on the basic Living-Longer-Stronger program. From the onset Larry was the most motivated of the group. He had an ideal combination of seriousness and humor. He was determined to do his best.

Strict Adherence

Many people involved in my programs do well for two weeks or so. Then, they are compelled to cheat on their dieting. A little more here, an extra bite there—unwarranted calories that slow down their fat losses. Not only did Larry not cheat, but he became the group's father confessor. If I scolded a member for a weekend lapse, Larry would provide a compassionate ear and offer helpful support. Such support not only assisted the member, but reinforced Larry.

The enthusiasm of the group combined with the program's synergy—the interaction and magnification of the eating plan, strength training, water drinking, walking after the evening meal, extra rest, and avoiding overstress—yielded awesome results. The group as a whole produced the most fat loss of any group I've ever worked with. And Larry Freedman dramatically shattered the individual record for fat loss.

LARRY'S ACCOMPLISHMENTS

In the 30 years that I've been supervising these diet and exercise programs, I've collectively trained more than 10,000 men. Larry accomplished more, and at a faster rate, than any of my other participants.

In six months, from April 4 through October 3, 1993, Larry lost 116½ pounds of fat and built 5½ pounds of muscle. He lost 15½ inches off his waist, 11 ¹/₈ inches off his hips, and 15 ³/₈ inches off his thighs. His body weight went from 306 to 195 pounds and his body fat decreased from 45 percent to 10.9 percent.

The amazing statistic, however, was that in his first six weeks, Larry lost 52 ¾ pounds of fat, for an average per week rate of 8.79 pounds, and an average daily rate of 1.26 pounds.

"I was ready for what this program had to offer," Larry said. "After the Christmas holidays, I was very depressed about my deplorable condition. I decided then that I was going to find the best way to get rid of my fat."

GUARANTEED FAT LOSS

Remember, Larry not only lost weight, but 100 percent of his weight loss was from his fat stores. How do I know this? Because I carefully measured his body

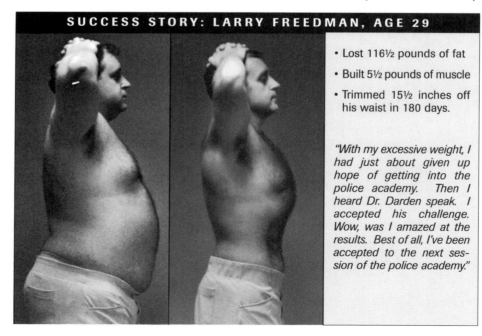

SUCCESS STORY: LARRY FREEDMAN, AGE 29

- Lost 116½ pounds of fat
- Built 5½ pounds of muscle
- Trimmed 15½ inches off his waist in 180 days.

"With my excessive weight, I had just about given up hope of getting into the police academy. Then I heard Dr. Darden speak. I accepted his challenge. Wow, was I amazed at the results. Best of all, I've been accepted to the next session of the police academy."

fat percentage before and after. Because I monitored all of his high-intensity work-outs. Because he lost more fat than he did weight, which meant that as he got stronger, he was building muscle.

Thus, the Living-Longer-Stronger program produced guaranteed fat loss within Larry's body. Instead of drawing fluids from his muscles, blood, and organs—which is typical of most weight-reduction plans—Larry burned calories from his adipose tissue, which is where he needed to lose them.

But that's not all. By building 5½ pounds of muscle, Larry increased his resting metabolic rate by approximately 275 calories per day. Losing fat and gain-ing muscle also improved dramatically the appearance of his physique, especially his waistline.

SELF-CONFIDENCE

The confidence that Larry now has in his body has transferred positively to his social life. "I used to spend most of my spare time eating, rarely leaving time to date," Larry said with a slight smile on his face. "As a result of my new physique and outlook, I now date in my spare time, rarely leaving time to eat."

Larry says he'll never be overfat again. I hope he's true to his pledge. It's been almost a year since Larry finished the program, and I frequently see him work-ing out at the Gainesville Health & Fitness Center. His body weight is still under 200 pounds and he looks better than ever.

Larry often introduces me to his friends with this comment: "Dr. Darden makes fat loss simple."

FAT LOSS MADE SIMPLE

Thanks, Larry. *Fat loss made simple* has a nice ring to it. But it's really only made simple if you have the necessary motivation and discipline, which obviously Larry had. And of course, there's the understanding and application of synergy, of which Larry took advantage.

I don't expect you to get the same results from the program as Larry did, unless you have more than 100 pounds to lose. But if you are typical—with from 20 to 30 pounds of excess fat—then with average application you can expect to lose from 3 to 4 pounds of fat per week for six weeks. With greater than average moti-vation and discipline, you can do even better.

33

BEFORE GETTING STARTED

There are some important steps to take before starting the Living-Longer-Stronger program. Devoting the necessary attention to each step will make it easier to reach your goal.

GET YOUR DOCTOR'S PERMISSION

Before you begin this program, be sure your doctor knows you plan to modify both your eating and exercising habits. Show him or her this book, so what is involved will be made clear. Your doctor will more than likely recommend a thorough physical examination, if you haven't had one in the last year.

DO BODY PART MEASUREMENTS

You and your partner can best do the measurements together. You'll need to wear a tight pair of swim trunks and have handy a plastic tape measure and a bathroom scale. Take and record the listed measurements on page 135.

Make sure you do all your measurements standing with your weight equally distributed on both feet. Apply the tape firmly, do not compress the skin, hold the tape parallel to the floor, and record the measurement to the nearest 1/8 inch.

SKIN-FOLD MEASURMENTS	Before	After
Right triceps	————	————
Right navel	————	————
Total	————	————
Percentage	————	————

Turn back to Chapter 23 and go through the skin-fold measurements to estimate your body fat percentage.

Full-length photographs of yourself in a tight bathing suit will prove meaningful as well. Stand against an uncluttered background with your hands on your head and your feet apart evenly. Pose to the camera from the front, side, and back.

BODY PART MEASUREMENTS			
	Before	**After**	**Difference**
Body weight	_____	_____	_____
Right upper arm (hanging in middle)	_____	_____	_____
Left upper arm (hanging in middle)	_____	_____	_____
Chest (at nipple level)	_____	_____	_____
Waist (at navel level)	_____	_____	_____
Hips (at largest protrusion with heels together)	_____	_____	_____
Right thigh (just below buttocks crease)	_____	_____	_____
Left thigh (just below buttocks crease)	_____	_____	_____

USE MEASURING SPOONS, CUPS, AND A SMALL SCALE

Most people overestimate one-half cup of orange juice, one tablespoon of raisins, or one ounce of mozzarella cheese. Such practices lead to sloppy recipe preparation, inaccurate calorie counting, and inefficient fat loss. It is important to become familiar with and correctly use measuring spoons, cups, and food scales.

Most of these items can be purchased inexpensively at your local department store or supermarket. With food scales, however, you'd be well advised to spend more money to purchase a battery-operated, digital scale instead of the less expensive, spring-loaded type.

PURCHASE A BOTTLE OF VITAMIN-MINERAL TABLETS

If you don't already take a vitamin-with-mineral tablet daily, then you should purchase an inexpensive bottle at your drug store or supermarket. Be certain no nutrient listed on the label exceeds 100 percent of the Recommended Dietary Allowances. High-potency supplements are not necessary. Take one multiple vitamin-with-minerals tablet each morning with breakfast.

Examine the Menus, Recipes, and Shopping Lists

Glance through the Living-Stronger-Longer menus, recipes, and shopping list in Chapter 35 for an overview of what you'll be eating during the six weeks. Your results will be more effective if you plan ahead.

Consider Giving Up Alcohol During the Program

If possible, give up alcoholic drinks entirely until you have reached your fat-loss goal. If you feel you must have a drink, limit your consumption to one light beer no more than three times per week. You'll see a light beer mentioned as an optional snack on some of the menus.

Most men found that one light beer didn't seem satisfying compared to their previous drinking habits. My advice to you is the same advice I gave to them: *avoid alcohol during the program.* Stick to more nutritious snacks to facilitate your results.

Avoid Intense Activity on Your Non-Exercise Days

Too much activity can be more harmful to your body than too little activity, especially when you're following a reduced-calorie diet. If you exercise intensely more than three times per week, your system soon reaches a state of overtraining. Fat losses and strength gains slow rather than accelerate. You eventually get the blahs, have little enthusiasm, and break your diet. At this point you are close to "burning the candle at both ends."

During your participation in the Living-Longer-Stronger diet and exercise program, it is to your advantage to keep your outside activities to a minimum. Naturally, you can continue with your normal work and responsibilities. Simply avoid vigorous activities such as running, skiing, racquetball, and basketball. Light recreational activities not carried to extremes are fine.

Once you reach your fat-loss goal, you can get involved in various strenuous sports and fitness activities if you wish.

FIND A PARTNER TO GO THROUGH THE PROGRAM WITH YOU

Although it is certainly possible to get great results going through the course by yourself, you'll lose more inches and pounds and build more muscle if you team up with a partner.

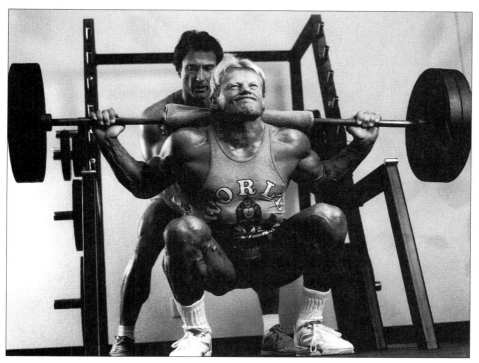

Frank Zane and Dave Draper (squatting), champion bodybuilders and both over 50 years of age, recognize the importance of training together.

34

THE LIVING-LONGER-STRONGER PROGRAM

Men and women in the United States spend more than $30 billion a year for products and services they hope will enable them to lose fat. Much of this money is wasted because the products and services are not based on sound, scientific facts.

Dr. Harold Cornacchia and Dr. Stephen Barrett, in their book, *Consumer Health: A Guide to Intelligent Decisions*, supply an excellent review of the popular scams in weight control. In this review, they note the following passage quoted from a publication of the American Medical Association:

> [These overweight people] will attend reducing clinics and join reducing programs. They will visit doctors who will write weight-reducing prescriptions for them and inject them with hormones. They will enter hospitals for fat-removing operations. They will get themselves hypnotized and psychoanalyzed individually and in groups. They will purchase books and pamphlets extolling the virtues of high-calorie diets, low-calorie diets; high fat, carbohy-drate and/or protein diets; low fat, carbohydrate and/or protein diets; grapefruit diets, water diets, drinking men's diets, organic food diets and sex-instead-of-supper diets. They will gulp down diet pills, blow on diet soups, chomp on diet cookies and chew on diet gum. Most of the time, for a variety of legitimate reasons, they will emerge in much the same condition as when they began: fat. And, much of the time, for a variety of illegitimate reasons, they will also emerge defrauded.

As I mentioned previously, there are more than 29,000 weight-loss plans, and the vast majority of them do not work. The Living-Longer-Stronger program *does* work. It works because it's based on tried-and-proven principles. It works because it requires your work.

That's right, *your work!* Nothing meaningful in your life has ever hap-pened to you that came as a result of quick and easy, has it? The work you will perform in the Living-Longer-Stronger program, however, is efficient, effective, and safe. It's the very best that science has to offer.

Almost every day for the next six weeks, you'll be applying to your lifestyle the following guidelines:

ADHERE TO A CARBOHYDRATE-RICH, DESCENDING-CALORIE EATING PLAN

Carbohydrates are your body's primary source of energy, as well as an important vehicle for the intake of many vitamins and minerals. Approximately 60 percent of your daily calories are from carbohydrate-rich foods on the Living-Longer-Stronger plan. The remaining 40 percent of the calories are equally divided between proteins and fats. The 60:20:20 ratio of carbohydrates, proteins, and fats is balanced and ideal for maximum fat loss. Furthermore, such a breakdown—with a slight modification or two—can be continued for a lifetime of healthy eating.

Many overfat men make the mistake of immediately reducing their calories from a typical 3,400 a day to 1,200 or fewer. Such a drastic cut in calories can cause at least three problems. First, after several days you may get an uncontrollable appetite, which causes you to break the diet. Second, a drastic reduction in calories may actually cause your body to fight to preserve its fat stores. Third, your body starts conserving energy and burns fewer and fewer calories. As a result, you'll have to reduce your food intake even more to keep losing. Such extremely low-calorie diets are doomed to failure.

I've found through my research that you can prevent all these problems by reducing your calories in a gradual manner. That's exactly what the Living-Longer-Stronger eating plan does.

You'll start with 1,500 calories per day, which means that you won't develop a ravenous appetite, nor will your body be stressed into its preservation stages. Quite the opposite will happen. Your body will become more efficient at burning fat. This is a major advantage of the descending-calorie plan.

Every two weeks, until the end of the sixth week, your calories are slightly reduced. Thus, during the fifth and sixth weeks, you are consuming 1,300 calories a day. This is as low as the descending-calorie diet ever goes for men.

The Living-Longer-Stronger diet offers daily menu selections that are low in saturated fat, cholesterol, and sodium. And you'll be pleasantly surprised by how little preparation is required.

EAT SMALLER MEALS MORE FREQUENTLY

You'll consume five small meals each day. You'll have a 300-calorie breakfast, a 300-calorie lunch, and a 500-calorie dinner. A mid-afternoon and a late-night snack, each from 100 to 200 calories, will round out the eating plan.

All the menus and recipes in the next chapter have been simplified. All you have to do is read and follow the easy-to-understand directions.

DRINK 128 TO 208 OUNCES OF COLD WATER EACH DAY

NUMBER OF OUNCES OF WATER PER DAY
Week 1 = 128
Week 2 = 144
Week 3 = 160
Week 4 = 176
Week 5 = 192
Week 6 = 208

Do not underestimate the importance of drinking plenty of cold water. Invariably the men who lose the most fat in six weeks are the most consistent with their water drinking.

You should begin your water drinking by consuming 1 gallon, or 128 ounces, a day for the first week. You then add 16 ounces a week until the end of the program, as indicated on the left.

During Week 6 you're consuming 208 ounces, or $1^5/8$ gallons, of water, a day. You may believe that it's impossible to drink that much water. It probably would be if you tried to gulp it down at one time. The secret is to spread it out, and drink 75 to 80 percent of the water before 5:00 P.M. Here's a weekly water-drinking schedule that many men find helpful:

WATER-DRINKING SCHEDULE						
Number Of 32-Ounce Bottles Per Day						
Time	**Wk 1**	**Wk 2**	**Wk 3**	**Wk 4**	**Wk 5**	**Wk 6**
7:00 A.M.						
	1.50	2.00	2.00	2.00	2.25	2.50
12:00 noon						
	1.50	1.50	2.00	2.00	2.25	2.50
5:00 P.M.						
	1.00	1.00	1.00	1.50	1.50	1.50
11:00 P.M.						
TOTAL:	**4.00**	**4.50**	**5.00**	**5.50**	**6.00**	**6.50**
Note: Drink 75-80 percent of water between 7:00 A.M. and 5:00 P.M.						

A 32-ounce, insulated plastic bottle with a straw makes the procedure easier to follow. Most men find they can consume more fluid with a straw than they can by drinking from a glass. A great way to keep up with your water drinking is to place rubber bands around the middle of the bottle equal to the number of bottles of water you are supposed to drink. Each time you finish 32 ounces, take off a rubber band.

APPLY STRENGTH TRAINING THREE TIMES PER WEEK

The Living-Longer-Stronger strength-training program stresses three non-consecutive-day, 25-minute workouts per week. As your dietary calories descend with each two weeks, the number of exercises gradually ascends. You perform only six exercises during weeks 1 and 2. You increase to eight exercises for the next two weeks. The final two weeks require a maximum of ten exercises.

WALK AFTER YOUR EVENING MEAL

You'll burn more calories if you take a leisurely walk after your evening meal each day. Remember, you should begin the walks within 15 minutes after the meal, and continue for 30 minutes only.

SLEEP AN EXTRA HOUR EACH NIGHT

Getting extra sleep will really help your fat-loss and muscle-building results. The best way to do this is to retire an hour earlier each night, but arise at the usual time each morning.

REMEMBER OTHER FAT-LOSS FACTS

Review often the facts in Chapter 30. It's to your advantage, for example, to sleep cool, avoid hot baths, practice good posture, brush your teeth often, and use color wisely. Little things, you should realize by now, can make a difference.

MILK AND DIGESTIVE PROBLEMS

Millions of people can't completely digest the sugar in milk. This problem is called lactose intolerance and can lead to bloating, excessive gas, abdominal cramping, and diarrhea. Research shows that lactose intolerance is prevalent in 8 percent of white Americans, 70 percent of African Americans, and 85 percent of Japanese. As men who have inherited this problem age, they gradually lose the ability to produce lactase, an enzyme that helps digest the lactose in milk and other dairy products.

What can you do if you have this problem, especially since dairy products are incorporated into the Living-Longer-Stronger eating plan?

There are a number of products, which you can find in your supermarket, that supply the enzyme lactase in pill or liquid form. Some of the brand names are DairyEase, Lactaid, Lactogest, and Lactrase. When consumed in the recommended dosages, any of these products can break down milk sugar and eliminate your previous digestive problems.

VEGETABLES: FRESH, FROZEN, OR CANNED?

There is a common belief that fresh vegetables are nutritionally superior to frozen or canned vegetables. While this belief may have been based on fact years ago, the sophisticated methods of food preservation applied in the 1990s reveal different conclusions.

In today's canning process, the vegetable is harvested at the proper time to assure optimal size, appearance, and nutritional value. The product is chilled immediately after picking and rushed to the factory. Once at the factory, it is washed and blanched and immediately processed by a short-term, high-temperature method. This cooking technique, followed by a very rapid cooling period, is the key to the superiority of industrial procedures over most home procedures. If the can is opened at home, it is necessary only to warm the food prior to serving. Furthermore, manufacturers now offer a wide variety of canned vegetables with *no salt added, no sugar added,* and *no preservatives added.*

In the freezing process, if vegetables are picked and then quick-frozen, the nutrient values are equal to or slightly higher than those of fresh vegetables.

Freshly harvested vegetables cooked immediately do not have significantly greater nutritional value than canned or frozen vegetables. Slow-cooking methods used at home often destroy more vitamins than are lost during the industrial processing. In fact, vegetables that have been poorly stored at the market may be less nutritious than those freshly picked from a home garden. Vegetables that are locally grown in season are frequently cheaper than commercially processed vegetables. But sometimes, even in season, fresh vegetables can be more expensive than canned or frozen ones.

From a nutritional viewpoint, it really doesn't matter whether you consume fresh, frozen, or canned vegetables. They are all rich in nutrients.

AVOID OVERSTRESS

Generally speaking, you want to stay clear of extremes. Send as many messages as you can to your body that everything is okay, standard, and tranquil. Do not get stressed out. Stay calm. Under such conditions, you will freely pull calories from your fat cells.

BE PATIENT

You are now well prepared to begin the Living-Longer-Stronger program. The next six weeks will make a difference in your life. Be patient. You can achieve your goals.

35
THE EATING PLAN: WEEKS 1–6

The menus in the Living-Longer-Stronger eating plan are designed for maximum fat-loss effectiveness and nutritional value. For best results, follow them exactly.

Every attempt has been made to keep current the popular brand names and calorie counts, which are listed in the menus. But as you probably know, products are sometimes changed or discontinued. If a listed product is not available in your area, for whatever reason, you'll have to substitute with something similar. Become a label reader at your supermarket. Don't be afraid to ask questions about the food products. Supermarket managers are usually very helpful. If they don't have the answers to your questions, they will find someone who does.

Each day you will choose a limited selection of foods for breakfast and lunch. I've found that most men can consume the same basic breakfast and the same basic lunch for months with little or no modification. Ample variety during your evening meal, however, will make daily eating interesting and enjoyable. Additionally, the eating plan includes a mid-afternoon and a late-night snack to keep your energy high and your hunger low.

Begin Week 1 on Monday and continue through Sunday. Week 2 is a repeat of Week 1. Calories for each food are noted in parentheses. A shopping list follows at the end of the chapter.

Remember, the eating plan for the next six weeks descends:

Weeks 1 & 2: 1,500 calories per day
Weeks 3 & 4: 1,400 calories per day
Weeks 5 & 6: 1,300 calories per day

You'll always have a 300-calorie breakfast, a 300-calorie lunch, and a 500-calorie dinner. With each two-week descent, only your snack calories will change: from 400 to 300 to 200 calories per day. For each of your five daily meals, you'll have at least three choices. Everything has been simplified so even the most kitchen-inept man can succeed. Very little cooking is required. All you have to do is read the following menus, select your food choices, and follow the directions. It's as simple as that.

MENUS FOR WEEKS 1 THROUGH 6

Breakfast = 300 calories. Choice of bagel, cereal, or shake.

1. **Bagel**

   1 plain bagel, Sara Lee Deli Style, frozen (190)

   1 ounce light cream cheese (60)

   ½ cup orange juice, fresh or frozen (55)

   Any beverage without calories, caffeine, or sodium, such as decaffeinated coffee or tea

2. **Cereal**

   1-ounce serving must equal 110 calories. Choice of one:

   > Kellogg's Cracklin' Oat Bran
   >
   > General Mills Clusters
   >
   > Post Honey Bunches of Oats
   >
   > Ralston Honey Almond Delight

   1 cup skim milk (90)

   1 cup orange juice (110)

   Noncaloric beverage

3. **Shake,** choice of one:

   Banana-Orange

   > 1 large banana (8¾ inches long) (100)
   >
   > ½ cup orange juice (55)
   >
   > ½ cup skim milk (45)
   >
   > 2 tablespoons wheat germ (66)
   >
   > 1 teaspoon safflower oil (42)
   >
   > 2 ice cubes (optional)
   >
   > Place ingredients in blender. Blend until smooth.

   Chocolate or Vanilla

   > 1 packet Carnation Instant Breakfast, Ultra Slim-Fast, or another diet shake powder that contains the appropriate calories (100)
   >
   > 1 cup skim milk (90)

½ banana (8¾ inches long) (50)

1 teaspoon safflower oil (42)

1 teaspoon Carnation Malted Milk powder (20)

2 ice cubes (optional)

Place ingredients in blender. Blend until smooth.

Lunch = 300 calories. Choice of one of three meals:

    1. Sandwich

        2 slices whole-wheat bread (140)

        2 teaspoons Promise *Ultra* Vegetable Oil Spread (24)

        2 ounces white meat (about 8 thin slices), chicken or turkey (80)

        1 ounce fat-free cheese (1½ slices) (50)

        Noncaloric beverage

    2. Soup

        choice of one:

            Healthy Choice Turkey Vegetable, 15-ounce can (220)

            Campbell's Healthy Request Hearty Chicken Rice, 16-ounce can (220)

        1 slice whole-wheat bread (70)

        1 teaspoon Promise *Ultra* Vegetable Oil Spread (12)

        Noncaloric beverage

    3. Chef Salad

        2 cups lettuce, chopped (20)

        2 ounces white meat, chicken or turkey (80)

        2 ounces fat-free cheese (100)

        4 slices tomato, chopped (28)

        1 tablespoon Italian fat-free dressing (6)

        1 slice whole-wheat bread (70)

        Noncaloric beverage

Mid-Afternoon Snack = 200 calories for Weeks 1 & 2, 150 calories for Weeks 3 & 4, 100 calories for Weeks 5 & 6. Combine for appropriate calories.

        1 large banana (8¾ inches long) (100)

        1 apple (3-inch diameter) (100)

        ½ cantaloupe (5-inch diameter) (94)

        5 dried prunes (100)

        1 ounce (2 small ½ ounce boxes) raisins (82)

        1 cup light, nonfat, flavored yogurt (100)

Dinner = 500 calories. Choice of one of three meals:

1. Tuna Salad Dinner

In a large bowl, mix the following:

    1 6-ounce can chunk light tuna in water (180)
    1 tablespoon Hellmann's Light Reduced-Calorie Mayonnaise (50)
    2 tablespoons Italian fat-free dressing (12)
    3 tablespoons sweet pickle relish (35)
    ½ cup whole kernel corn, canned, no salt added (45)

½ cup sliced white potatoes, canned (45)

2 slices whole-wheat bread (140)

Noncaloric beverage

2. Steak Dinner

3 ounces lean sirloin, broiled (176)

½ cup sweet peas, canned, no salt added (60)

½ cup beets, canned (35)

2 slices whole-wheat bread (140)

1 teaspoon Promise *Ultra* Vegetable Oil Spread (12)

1 cup skim milk (90)

Noncaloric beverage

3. Frozen Microwave Dinner

Choose one of five recommended meals:

Glazed Chicken Dinner, Lean Cuisine (240)

2 slices whole-wheat bread (140)

2 teaspoons Promise *Ultra* Vegetable Oil Spread (24)

1 cup skim milk (90)

Noncaloric beverage

Lasagna with Meat Sauce, Lean Cuisine (270)

2 slices whole-wheat bread (140)

1 cup skim milk (90)

Noncaloric beverage

Macaroni and Cheese, Healthy Choice (290)

2 slices whole-wheat bread (140)

1 teaspoon Promise *Ultra* Vegetable Oil Spread (12)

²/₃ cup skim milk (60)
Noncaloric beverage

Shrimp & Vegetable Maria, Healthy Choice (260)
2 slices whole-wheat bread (140)
3 teaspoons Promise *Ultra* Vegetable Oil Spread (36)
²/₃ cup skim milk (60)
Noncaloric beverage

Country Inn Roast Turkey Classic, Healthy Choice (250)
2 slices whole-wheat bread (140)
2 teaspoons Promise *Ultra* Vegetable Oil Spread (24)
1 cup skim milk (90)
Noncaloric beverage

Late Night Snack = 200 calories for Weeks 1 & 2, 150 calories for Weeks 3 & 4, and 100 calories for Weeks 5 & 6. Combine for appropriate calories. See Mid-Afternoon Snack plus the following:

   1 cup ice milk or low-fat frozen yogurt (100)
   12 ounces light beer (100)
   2 cups light, microwave popcorn (100)

SHOPPING LIST

   Quantities needed for listed items will depend on your specific selections. Review your choices and adjust the shopping list accordingly. It may be helpful for you to photocopy this list each week before doing your shopping. Also, a photocopy of the eating plan chart at the end of this chapter will assist you.

LIVING-LONGER-STRONGER SHOPPING LIST

Staples

orange juice

skim milk

whole-wheat bread

Promise *Ultra* Vegetable Oil Spread

Italian fat-free dressing

safflower oil

Hellman's Light Reduced-Calorie Mayonnaise

sweet pickle relish

noncaloric beverages (tea, coffee, diet soft drinks, water)

Grains

bagels, Sara Lee Deli Style, frozen

cereals, 1-ounce serving must equal 110 calories

> Kellogg's Cracklin' Oat Bran
>
> General Mills Clusters
>
> Post Honey Bunches of Oats
>
> Ralston Honey Almond Delight

wheat germ

malted milk powder

popcorn, microwave light

light beer

Fruits

bananas, large (8¾ inches long)

apples (3-inch diameter)

cantaloupes (5-inch diameter)

dried prunes

raisins

Vegetables

lettuce

tomatoes

whole kernel corn, canned, no salt added

sweet peas, canned, no salt added

sliced white potatoes, canned

cut beets, canned

Dairy

yogurt, light nonfat

cream cheese, light

cheese, fat-free

ice milk or low-fat frozen yogurt

Carnation Instant Breakfast packets

Ultra Slim-Fast packets

Meat, Poultry, Fish, and Entrees

chicken, thin sliced

turkey, thin sliced

tuna, canned chunk light in water

sirloin steak, lean

canned soup

> Healthy Choice Turkey Vegetable
>
> Campbell's Healthy Request Hearty Chicken Rice

frozen microwave dinners or entrees

> Lean Cuisine Glazed Chicken Dinner
>
> Lean Cuisine Lasagna with Meat Sauce
>
> Healthy Choice Macaroni and Cheese
>
> Healthy Choice Shrimp & Vegetable Maria
>
> Healthy Choice Country Inn Roast Turkey Classic

LIVING-LONGER-STRONGER EATING PLAN

Name _____

Date _____

Circle the appropriate week, Calorie Level, and Entree

Week	1	2	3	4	5	6
Calorie Level	1500		1400		1300	

Breakfast

Weeks 1-2 = 300 Calories
Weeks 3-4 = 300 Calories
Weeks 5-6 = 300 Calories

One Choice = 300 Calories

Bagel

Cracklin' Oat Bran

Clusters

Honey Bunches of Oats

Honey Almond Delight

Banana-Orange Shake

Chocolate Shake

Vanilla Shake

Lunch

Weeks 1-2 = 300 Calories
Weeks 3-4 = 300 Calories
Weeks 5-6 = 300 Calories

One Choice = 300 Calories

Chicken Sandwich

Turkey Sandwich

Turkey Vegetable Soup

Chicken Rice Soup

Chicken Chef Salad

Turkey Chef Salad

Mid-day Snack

Weeks 1-2 = 200 Calories
Weeks 3-4 = 150 Calories
Weeks 5-6 = 100 Calories

One Choice = 100 Calories

Banana

Apple

Cantaloupe

Prunes

Raisins

Yogurt

Dinner

Weeks 1-2 = 500 Calories
Weeks 3-4 = 500 Calories
Weeks 5-6 = 500 Calories

One Choice = 500 Calories

Tuna Salad

Steak

Glazed Chicken

Lasagna

Macaroni

Shrimp

Turkey

Late-night Snack

Weeks 1-2 = 200 Calories
Weeks 3-4 = 150 Calories
Weeks 5-6 = 100 Calories

One Choice = 100 Calories

Banana

Apple

Cantaloupe

Prunes

Raisins

Yogurt

Ice Milk

Light Beer

Popcorn

36

THE EXERCISE ROUTINE:
WEEKS 1–6

Strength-training exercise is an important component of the Living-Longer-Stronger program. From previous chapters, you should be convinced that strength training is the best type of activity for fat loss. Larger, stronger muscles aid fat loss by consuming more calories at work and at rest.

PRECISION BASICS

Examine first: Spend several minutes looking over the exercises in this chapter. Read the directions carefully to get an idea of the routine. Practice will perfect your form and maximize results.

Choose between machines and barbells: If you train at home, you'll probably use barbells and dumbbells. If you exercise at a commercial fitness center or gym, you'll probably have access to both machines and free weights. Most of the men who have been through the six-week program used machines. Most machines have obvious advantages, as I explained in an earlier chapter. I'd recommend that you use machines *or* free weights for the six-week program, as opposed to intermingling them.

Select the appropriate resistance: Initially it's important that you learn how to perform each exercise correctly. You'll learn better if the resistance is not too heavy and not too light. Of course, what's light for you may be heavy for someone else, so it would be useless to list starting poundages. Try to select a moderate weight at first, something you can do easily for 8 repetitions. After a week or so, increase the resistance so that 8 repetitions are challenging.

Control your movements: Rushing through each exercise diminishes results and can cause injury. Do each repetition slowly, smoothly, and intensely. Each exercise should take approximately 4 seconds on the lifting and 4 seconds on the lowering.

Emphasize breathing: Try not to hold your breath during any exercise.

Keep your mouth open and breathe. When the movement gets difficult, purse your lips and work on blowing out.

Count the repetitions: Start with 8 repetitions on each exercise. Add repetitions with each workout until 12 or more can be performed in correct form. Increase the resistance by 5 percent at the next workout, and continue in your progression.

Focus your attention: Proper exercise is both physical and mental. Direct your attention to the muscles you're working, and your results will improve. If it's a trunk curl, for example, focus on the front abdominals. Try to see them contracting in your mind each time you lift and lower. The effort will make a difference.

Expect some soreness: Soreness in exercised body parts is an indication that you've stretched and contracted little-used muscles. Expect some tenderness after your first workout. Your second workout will ease the soreness, and it should be gone by your third exercise session.

MACHINE ROUTINES

For these routines, you'll need access to a basic set of exercise machines—such as Nautilus, MedX, Cybex, BodyMaster, or Hammer—which are found in fitness centers throughout the United States. The following routines involve three non-consecutive-day—usually Monday, Wednesday, Friday—workouts per week. Perform six exercises during Weeks 1 and 2, eight exercises for the middle two weeks, and ten during Weeks 5 and 6.

MACHINE ROUTINES		
Weeks 1 & 2	**Weeks 3 & 4**	**Weeks 5 & 6**
1. Leg Curl	1. Leg Curl	1. Leg Curl
2. Leg Extension	2. Leg Extension	2. Leg Extension
3. Lateral Raise	3. Lateral Raise	3. Leg Press*
4. Pullover	4. Pullover	4. Lateral Raise
5. Bench Press	5. Bench Press	5. Pullover
6. Abdominal	6. Biceps Curl*	6. Bench Press
	7. Lower Back*	7. Biceps Curl
	8. Abdominal	8. Triceps Extension*
		9. Lower Back
* Indicates new exercise		10. Abdominal

DESCRIPTION OF EACH MACHINE EXERCISE

Leg Curl Machine

Muscles worked: The leg curl machine works the hamstrings, which are located on the back of your thighs. Composed of three large muscles, the major function of the hamstrings is to bend your legs. Although some leg curl machines are performed from a seated position, most are done by lying prone. The instructions below are for the prone leg curl machine.

Contracted position

Starting position: Lie face down on the machine. Move your feet under the roller pads, with your knees just over the edge of the bench. Place your chin on a small pad, or turn your face to either side, whichever is more comfortable for you. Grasp the handles to keep your upper body from moving.

Exercise performance: Curl your legs smoothly in 4 seconds and try to touch your heels to your buttocks. Lift your hips slightly to increase your range of movement. Do *not* try to keep your front hips flat against the pad. Pause briefly in the contracted position. Lower the resistance slowly in 4 seconds. Repeat for maximum repetitions. If you can do 12 or more repetitions, increase the resistance by 5 percent at your next workout.

Training tips: Keep your toes pointed toward your knees throughout the movement. Come to a complete stop in the contracted position.

Leg Extension Machine

Contracted position

Muscles worked: The leg extension machine involves the quadriceps, the largest muscles at the front of your thighs. The tendons of these four muscles cross your knee joints and attach to your leg bones. Contraction of the quadriceps causes your knees to extend and your legs to straighten. Exercising these large muscles builds, strengthens, and tightens the front of your thighs and improves the structural integrity of your knees.

Starting position: Sit in the machine. Place your feet behind the roller pads. Adjust the seat back to a comfortable position. Fasten the seat belt across your hips. Keep your head and shoulders against the seat back. Grasp the handles lightly.

Exercise performance: Straighten both legs smoothly in 4 seconds. Pause briefly in the top position. Lower the resistance slowly in 4 seconds. Repeat for maximum repetitions.

Training tips: Concentrate on isolating your quadriceps by moving the resistance smoothly and slowly. Do not bounce in and out of the top position. Do not stop and rest in the bottom position. Do not lean your torso forward or arch your back excessively. Practice relaxing your neck and face during the last repetitions.

Lateral Raise Machine

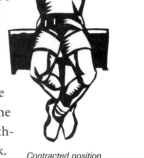

Contracted position

Muscles worked: The lateral raise provides direct exercise for the deltoids. The deltoids are triangle-shaped muscles that drape over your shoulders with one angle pointing down your arm and the other two bending around your shoulder to the front and rear. Stronger deltoids broaden your shoulders. They also help prevent or alleviate slumped or rounded posture.

Starting position: Sit facing out in the machine. Adjust the seat until your shoulder joints are in line with the axes of rotation of the machine's movement arms. Fasten the seat belt. Pull your knees together and cross your ankles. Grasp the handles lightly and pull back. Make sure your upper arms are approximately parallel to your torso.

Exercise performance: Raise your elbows smoothly to about ear level. Pause briefly in the top position. Lower your elbows and upper arms slowly to your sides. Repeat for maximum repetitions.

Training tips: Lead with your elbows, not your hands. Do not allow your upper arms to move forward gradually. Keep them back in line with your upper body.

Pullover Machine

Muscles worked: The pullover machine involves the largest and strongest muscles of your upper body, the latissimus dorsi. These muscles join to the lower part of your spine and sweep up both sides of your back to your armpits, where they are attached to your upper arm bones. The latissimus dorsi enable your upper arms to rotate from an overhead position down to your waist. Strengthening these muscles will assist you in all arm-movement activities, such as swinging a racquet or a golf club, throwing a ball, swimming, and pulling with your arms. When significantly developed, the latissimus dorsi muscles will improve your upper back's strength and width, and your overall posture.

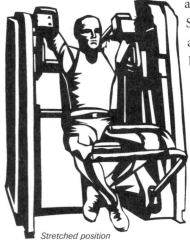
Stretched position

Starting position: Adjust the seat so your shoulder joints are in line with the movement arm's axes of rotation. Assume an erect position and fasten the seat belt tightly around your hips. Leg press the foot pedal until the elbow pads are brought to about chin level. Place your elbows on the pads. Your hands should be open and resting on the bar.

Exercise performance: Remove your feet from the foot pedal and slowly rotate your elbows back until a comfortable stretch is felt. Rotate your elbows forward and downward until the bar touches your midsection. Pause. Return slowly to the stretched position. Stretch. Repeat for maximum repetitions. If you can do 12 or more repetitions, increase the resistance by 5 percent at your next workout.

Training tips: Do not arch your back excessively in the stretched position. Do not lean your torso forward excessively in the contracted position. Do not grip with your hands. Do not push with your head against the seat back.

Bench Press Machine

Muscles worked: The bench press machine supplies movement around your shoulders and elbows. The primary muscles worked are the pectoralis major, deltoid, and triceps. Developing your chest and shoulder muscles prevents much of the flat, bony look that many men have to their upper torso. Some chest press machines are performed seated, while others are done while lying flat on a bench. The one I describe below is done on a bench in a supine position.

Starting position: Lie face up on the bench

Top position

with the handles beside your chest. Stabilize your body by placing your feet flat on the floor or on a raised step. Grasp the handles lightly.

Exercise performance: Press the handles upward smoothly in 4 seconds. Do not jam into a forceful lockout with your elbows. Lower the handles slowly to the bottom in 4 seconds. Repeat for maximum repetitions.

Training tips: Do not move your hips during the pressing action. Do not arch your back excessively.

Abdominal Machine

Muscles worked: The abdominal machine stresses the rectus abdominis muscles of your front waist. The function of the rectus abdominis is to enable your rib cage and pelvic girdle to move close together. Keeping this muscle group strong helps to improve a flabby belly and a protruding waistline. Many different abdominal machines are being manufactured today. The one I discuss below is the latest version (Next Generation) made by Nautilus.

Starting position: Adjust the seat so your navel aligns with the red dot on the side of the machine. Fasten the set belt across your hips. Cross your ankles. Place your elbows on the pads and grasp the handles lightly.

Exercise performance: Pull with your elbows and shorten the distance between your lower ribs and pelvis. Do not try to pivot around your hips. Pause in the contracted position. Return slowly to the starting position. Repeat for maximum repetitions.

Training tips: Keep your shoulders against the set back throughout the entire movement. Do not jut your chin forward at the start. Do not try to do a sit-up on this machine. Do not move quickly. Do not pull excessively with your arms. Pull with your midsection.

Contracted position

Biceps Curl Machine

Muscles worked: This machine acts on the biceps, the prominent muscles on the front of your upper arms. One function of your biceps is bending your arm, and your arms bend hundreds of times each day as you go about your normal activities.

Starting position: Stand and place your elbows in line with the axes of the machine's movement arms. Grasp the handles lightly. Bend your arms to 90

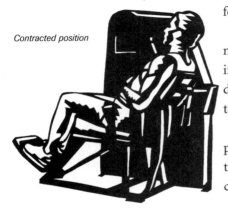

Starting position

degrees and be seated. Lower your hands until your arms are straight. Your shoulders should be stable and secure. If not, relax your arms and readjust the seat.

Exercise performance: Curl both handles to the contracted position. Your thumbs should almost touch your shoulders. Pause. Lower slowly to the starting position. Repeat for maximum repetitions.

Training tips: Do not allow your elbows to slide out of position. They should remain in line with the axes of rotation. Do not raise and lower your shoulders during the exercise. Keep your shoulders stable. Make sure your seat is not too low, as this can cause too much stress on your elbows. Keep your wrists firm during the movement.

Lower Back Machine

Muscles worked: Since the lower back is so prone to injury, a more thorough discussion is necessary for this machine and the muscles involved. Many lower back machines on the market actually work your hips and thighs more than your lower back. To successfully isolate your lower back muscles, your pelvis must be rigidly secured. Only MedX and Nautilus make machines that accomplish this goal.

The primary muscles of your lower back are the erector spinae. These muscles lie on both sides of your spinal column, and when they contract they extend your torso backward. Extending the torso backward provides safe exercise for a troublesome area of the body.

Contracted position

Lower back problems are caused by at least three major conditions: sudden compression forces, sudden twisting movements combined with compression forces, and sudden movements combined with compression forces that lead to excessive arching of the back.

The lower back machine does *not* supply sudden compression forces to your spine. The resistance transferred by the movement arm is always perpendicular to your spinal column. Thus, any dangerous vertical loading is eliminated.

The lower back machine does *not* allow you to twist

while performing the exercise. The movement is backward and forward, with no twisting or grinding motions.

The lower back exercise is *not* performed suddenly in a ballistic manner. The movements are always done in a slow, smooth manner. Furthermore, the limited range of movement built into the machine and the seat belts prevent excessive arching of the back.

A strong lower back will improve your posture and carriage. It will assist your performance in most movement activities. Stronger muscles will also keep back injury from becoming a chronic problem.

If you have existing lower back pain, or a past history of lower back pain, consult with your physician before using this machine.

Starting position: Sit in the machine. Make sure your hips are well back in the seat. Adjust the footrest so your thighs are slightly elevated off the seat bottom. (Some smaller men may require an extra pad to sit on.) Fasten both seat belts securely across your hips and thighs. Put your hands across your waist and interlace your fingers.

Exercise performance: Extend your torso backward smoothly by rotating your lower back around the edge of the seat back. Pause in the contracted position. Return slowly to the starting position. Repeat for 8 to 12 repetitions.

Training tips: Slow, smooth movement is especially important in this machine. Do not ever jerk or bounce at the start, or the end, of the range of motion. Keep your head in one stable position throughout.

Leg Press Machine

Muscles worked: The leg press is a very demanding machine. It is demanding because it involves your lower body's largest muscles: erector spinae, gluteus maximus, quadriceps, hamstrings, and gastrocnemius.

Starting position: Adjust the seat back to a comfortable position. Crank the seat carriage until your knees, with your feet in the proper position on the movement arm, are near your chest. The closer the seat is to the movement arm, the longer the range of motion and the more productive the exercise. Both seat back and seat carriage should be adjusted to same position each time you do the exercise. Sit in the machine with your feet

Starting position

placed evenly on the foot pedal or movement arm. Grasp lightly the handles by your hips.

Exercise performance: Push with your feet and straighten both legs smoothly in 4 seconds. Do not lock your knees. Keep them bent slightly. Lower the weight slowly in 4 seconds. Repeat for maximum repetitions.

Training tips: Work diligently on keeping your movement continuous. Try not to stop at either the start or the extended position. Practice keeping your face and neck relaxed.

Triceps Extension Machine

Muscles worked: The triceps are on the back side of your upper arms. The major function of the triceps is to straighten your elbows. Strengthening your triceps will allow you to make better use of your arms in many daily tasks and fitness activities.

Mid-range position

Starting position: Adjust the seat so that your shoulders are at a level slightly lower than your elbows. Place the sides of your hands on the movement arms and your elbows on the pad in line with the axes of the movement arms.

Exercise performance: Straighten both arms into the contracted position. Pause. Lower slowly to the stretched position. Your thumbs should be near your shoulders. Repeat for maximum repetitions. If you can do 12 or more repetitions, increase the resistance by 5 percent at your next workout.

Training tips: Do not bounce in and out of the contracted position. Do not raise your shoulders when your arms are straightening. Do not move your head forward.

BARBELL-DUMBBELL ROUTINES

Following are the recommended free-weight routines.

BARBELL-DUMBBELL ROUTINES		
Weeks 1 & 2	**Weeks 3 & 4**	**Weeks 5 & 6**
1. Squat with Barbell	1. Squat with Barbell	1. Squat with Barbell
2. Prone Back Raise	2. Prone Back Raise	2. Prone Back Raise
3. Lateral Raise with Dumbbells	3. Stiff-Legged Deadlift with Barbell*	3. Stiff-Legged Deadlift with Barbell
4. Pullover with Dumbbell	4. Lateral Raise with Dumbbells	4. One-Legged Calf Raise with Dumbbell*
5. Bench Press with Barbell	5. Pullover with Dumbbell	5. Lateral Raise with Dumbbells
6. Trunk Curl	6. Bench Press with Barbell	6. Pullover with Dumbbell
	7. Biceps Curl with Barbell*	7. Bench Press with Barbell
	8. Trunk Curl	8. Biceps Curl with Barbell
		9. Triceps Extension with Dumbbell*
* Indicates new exercise		10. Trunk Curl

DESCRIPTION OF EACH FREE-WEIGHT EXERCISE

Squat with Barbell

Muscles worked: The squat primarily stresses your gluteus maximus, quadriceps, hamstrings, and erector spinae muscles. Secondary emphasis is placed on the smaller muscles of your upper back, midsection, and calves.

Starting position: Place a barbell on a squat rack and load it with the appropriate amount of weight. Position the bar behind your neck across your trapezius muscles and hold it in place with your hands. If the bar cuts into your skin, pad it lightly by wrapping a towel around the knurl. Straighten your legs to lift the bar off the rack and move back one step. Place your feet shoulder-width apart, toes angled slightly outward. Keep your upper body muscles rigid and your torso upright during the exercise. It also helps if you focus on a spot on the wall at eye level as you do the movement.

Exercise performance: Bend your hips and knees and smoothly descend to a position where your hamstrings firmly come in contact with your calves. Without bouncing, and without stopping in the bottom position, slowly make the turnaround from down to up. Smoothly lift the barbell back almost to the top position. Do not lock your legs. Keep a bend of approximately 15 degrees in your knees. Repeat for maximum repetitions.

Mid-range position

Training tips: It's important that you don't allow your torso to bend forward as you rise out of the bottom position. You'll find it easier to perform a repetition with this cheating technique, but it takes stress from your thighs and places potentially harmful force on your lower back. As a safety measure, it is also a good idea to use spotters during the squat.

Prone Back Raise

Muscles worked: This exercise stresses your erector spinae and gluteus maximus muscles.

Starting position: If you work out in a gym that has a special bench for the back raise, use it. If not, you'll have to get a partner to assist you in this exercise. Lie face down, lengthwise on a bench. Support the lower half of your body by having your navel even with the edge of the bench. Your partner stands behind and holds your feet and legs down. Place your hands behind your neck.

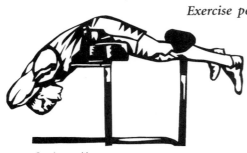

Exercise performance: Lean forward and bend at your waist. Raise your torso smoothly backward. There should be a slight arch in your back in the top position. Pause. Lower slowly. Repeat for 8 to 12 repetitions.

Training tips: Make sure your navel does not slide forward. Keep it at the edge of the bench. Do not move your head during the movement. Keep it in one position.

Starting position

Lateral Raise with Dumbbells

Muscles worked: The lateral raise involves the deltoids.

Starting position: Grasp a dumbbell in each hand and stand. Lock your elbows and wrists and keep them locked throughout the exercise. All the action should occur around your shoulder joints.

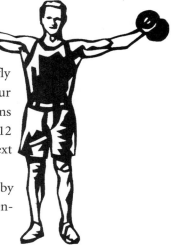

Contracted position

Exercise performance: Raise your arms sideways. Pause briefly when the dumbbells are slightly above the horizontal. Make sure your palms are facing down and your elbows are straight. Lower your arms slowly to your sides. Repeat for maximum repetitions. If you can do 12 or more repetitions, increase the resistance by 5 percent at your next workout.

Training tips: Resist the temptation to cheat on this exercise by leaning forward, bringing the dumbbells together, and using momentum to initiate the movement at the bottom.

Pullover with Dumbbell

Muscles worked: This exercise involves your latissimus dorsi muscles. It also stretches your rib cage.

Starting position: Lie crossways on a bench with your shoulders in contact with the bench and your head and lower body relaxed and off the bench. Hold a dumbbell on one end in both hands and position it over your chest with your arms straight.

Exercise performance: Take a deep breath and lower the dumbbell smoothly behind your head. Stretch and raise the dumbbell slowly to the over-chest position. Repeat for maximum repetitions.

Training tips: The emphasis in this exercise is on the stretching that occurs in the bottom position. Stretching is stressed more when your arms are straight. With too heavy a weight you'll probably have to bend your arms. Lighten the resistance and practice stretching with your arms straight. You'll feel the effect much more in your rib cage.

Starting position

Bench Press with Barbell

Muscles worked: A favorite exercise of many bodybuilders, the bench press stresses the pectorals, deltoids, and triceps.

Starting position: Load a barbell resting on the rack at the head end of a flat exercise bench. Lie on the bench with your shoulders under the barbell and your feet in a stable position on the floor. Grasp the barbell with your hands shoulder-width apart. Straighten your arms to bring the barbell to a supported position directly above your shoulders.

Bottom position

Exercise performance: Lower the barbell smoothly to your chest. Without bouncing the bar off your chest, press the weight until your arms are almost straight. Keep a slight bend in your elbows in the top position. Repeat for maximum repetitions.

Training tips: Many bodybuilders experiment on the bench press by using wider grips. This is usually a mistake. Since the function of your chest muscles is to move your upper arms across your torso, spacing your hands wider than your shoulders actually shortens your range of movement. Rather than working more of your chest muscles, you're working less of them. For best results on the bench press, keep your hands shoulder-width apart. It's also a good idea to have a person spot you in case you get in trouble with the weight.

Trunk Curl

Muscles worked: This exercise is performed on the floor and acts on the rectus abdominis and oblique muscles.

Starting position: Lie face up on the floor with your hands behind your head. Keep your chin tucked into your chest. Bring your heels up close to your buttocks and spread your knees. Do not anchor your feet under anything, and don't have a partner hold your knees down. Anchoring your feet brings into action your hip flexors more than your abdominals.

Contracted position

Exercise performance: Curl your shoulders smoothly toward your hips. Only one-third of a standard sit-up can be performed in this manner. When you do this movement correctly, you will feel a powerful contraction in your rectus abdominis muscles. Pause in the contracted position. Lower your shoulders to the floor. Repeat for maximum repetitions.

Training tips: Do not arch your lumbar spine excessively at the start. Keep the movement slow and steady. When 12 or more repetitions of the trunk curl can be accomplished in proper form, add a light barbell plate across your chest.

Stiff-Legged Deadlift with Barbell

Muscles worked: The deadlift involves the erector spinae, gluteus maximus, and hamstrings.

Starting position: Even though this exercise is called a stiff-legged deadlift, it should be performed with a slight bend in your knees. This protects the vertebrae of your lower back. Grasp the barbell with one hand under and the other hand over. Your feet should be under the bar. Bend your knees and stand with the barbell.

Stretched position

Exercise performance: Lower the barbell slowly down your thighs toward the floor. Keep a slight bend in your knees. Lift the barbell smoothly back to an almost erect position. Repeat for 8 to 12 repetitions.

Training tips: Ease into the stiff-legged deadlift, especially if you have any problems or tenderness in your lower back. For several weeks, use a light weight and do not go to momentary muscular failure. Move extra slowly in and out of the bottom position.

Biceps Curl with Barbell

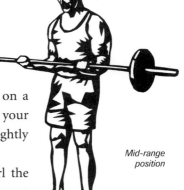

Muscles worked: The curl acts on the biceps of your upper arm.

Starting position: Take a shoulder-width underhand grip on a barbell and stand. Anchor your elbows firmly against the sides of your waist and keep them there throughout the exercise. Lean forward slightly with your shoulders.

Mid-range position

Exercise performance: Look down at your hands and curl the weight smoothly in 4 seconds. Pause in the top position, but do not move your elbows forward. Keep your hands in front of your elbows. Lower the bar slowly in 4 seconds. Again, keep your elbows stable against your sides for maximum repetitions.

Training tips: Maximize your biceps stimulation by minimizing your body sway. Do not lean forward excessively. Do not lean backward. Do not move your head. Concentrate on your breathing and keep the repetitions slow, smooth, and strict.

One-Legged Calf Raise with Dumbbell

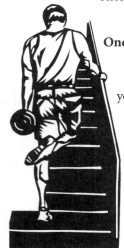

Muscles worked: The one-legged calf raise is one of the best exercises for your gastrocnemius and soleus muscles.

Starting position: A sturdy four-inch block of wood or some other four-inch-high platform is necessary for this movement. Stand with a light dumbbell in your left hand. Place the ball of your left foot on the block. Use your right hand to hold on to something to stabilize your body.

Exercise performance: Raise and lower your left heel in a smooth, slow style, while keeping your left knee locked. Concentrate on contracting at the top and stretching at the bottom. When your left calf is exhausted, switch the dumbbell to your right hand and repeat the procedure for your right calf.

Contracted position for left calf

Training tips: Since the range of motion in this exercise is short, it is especially important to move slowly and pause briefly at each turnaround. If you are performing this exercise by standing on a block of wood, make sure it is stable.

Triceps Extension with Dumbbell

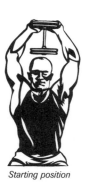

Muscles worked: This exercise isolates the triceps of your upper arms.

Starting position: Hold a dumbbell at one end with both hands. Press the dumbbell overhead. Your elbows should be pointed up.

Exercise performance: Bend your elbows and slowly lower the dumbbell behind your neck. Do not move your elbows. Only your forearms and hands should move. Press the dumbbell smoothly back to the starting position. Repeat for maximum repetitions.

Training tips: In the bottom position of this exercise, the triceps is stretched across two joints. Thus, it is vulnerable to strains. Make sure this does not occur by keeping your lower turnarounds smooth and slow.

Starting position

CHARTING YOUR PROGRESS

It's important to keep accurate records of all your workouts. The following routine chart has room for ten exercises with space to the right to note your resistance and repetitions for the six workouts that comprise each two-week segment.

Make three photocopies of this page for your six-week program. Fill in the blanks at the top of each copy with your name and the appropriate weeks. List your exercises for each two-week segment in the left column. Now, you're ready to progress through the routines.

LIVING-LONGER-STRONGER EXERCISE ROUTINE						
Name_____ Weeks_____						
Exercise / Date / **Body Weight**						
1.						
2.						
3.						
4.						
5.						
6.						
7.						
8.						
9.						
10.						

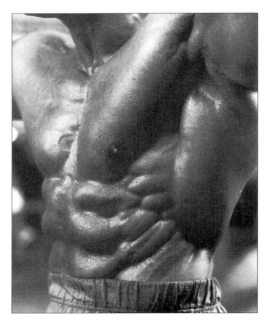

Getting—and maintaining—a lean waist requires disciplined actions, as well as a knowledge of how to anticipate and deal with problems.

37
TROUBLESHOOTING

During the first several weeks or months of any new eating and exercising plan, certain situations may arise that cause trouble. For example, how do you deal with eating out? Or how about those holiday parties? Or that summer vacation? The following troubleshooting guide will help you deal with these and other challenges to sustaining your program.

EATING OUT ON THE LIVING-LONGER-STRONGER DIET

In today's health- and fitness-conscious society, virtually no restaurant is going to be surprised by or unprepared to accommodate special dietary requests.

The problem is not with the eating establishment, but with knowing how to order in a specific manner. Here are the best guidelines to use when ordering your meal:

- *Leave the menu unopened.* The purpose of the menu is to entice you to spend big, and restaurants really know how to sell the sizzle.

- *Ask the waiter what kind of fresh fish is available.* Though chicken is as acceptable as fish, you are better off with fish, which is always prepared to order. Because of its lengthier preparation time, chicken is usually partially prepared earlier in the day with various marinades and sauces.

- *Choose a white fish* and have it baked, steamed, or broiled, with nothing on it.

- *Inquire about vegetables* and select two with nothing added. A plain baked potato is always available. Other good choices are broccoli, cauliflower, and carrots.

- *Order a simple green salad* without such garnishes as croutons or bacon bits. Lemon juice, vinegar, or low-calorie dressing is preferable to any creamy or oily dressings.

- *Request a large pitcher of ice water* to be placed on your table. Drink freely before, during, and after your meal.

- *Have caffeine-free coffee or tea* for dessert, or at most, some fruit, such as strawberries or raspberries.

- *Be assertive.* Diet-conscious diners are changing restaurants by demanding a greater variety of lower-calorie foods. You'll find diet sodas, sugar and salt substitutes, caffeine-free coffee and tea, whole-grain breads, fresh fruits and vegetables, and nonfat salad dressings in practically any restaurant you visit.

- *Be very specific with your order.* Double-check to make sure that your waiter understands exactly what you want.

COMBATING HOLIDAY CALORIES

The holiday season brings the office party, the family get-together, the reunion with out-of-town friends. There are the NFL playoffs and the college bowl games. Also on the schedule is this or that organization's holiday bash. A calorie-consumption catastrophe is under way.

But it doesn't have to be. If you don't want to begin the new year by having your wardrobe altered a size or two larger, devise your plan of defense now.

When you're the host, serve low-calorie meals and snacks and offer more activities than just sitting and eating. Still, what happens under your own roof isn't the big problem.

You'll be eating and drinking more often at locations out of your direct control. Here are four important steps to take.

- *Plan ahead, eat ahead.* If the festivity includes dinner, find out what is on the menu. If there are not enough good choices, or if dinner is served well past your normal mealtime, eat at home. Budget 100 to 200 calories for some polite eating at the party.

- *Limit alcohol intake.* Alcohol is one of the most calorie-dense foods. Alcohol also tends to be accompanied with munchies galore. As judgment blurs, there's more to drink, more munchies. Social drinking can produce a quantum leap in your daily calorie intake. Couldn't you still enjoy your party if you halved your alcohol intake?

First, never drink alcohol when you're thirsty. Quench your thirst with water. If you're having mixed drinks, drink the mixer alone every other round.

- *Say "no" firmly but gracefully.* You'll flatter the hostess—and avoid eating her mega-calorie offering—by telling her how delicious it looks and requesting the recipe. But you're unable to eat right now, darn it. You must be firm. This won't be easy because others will tempt you and even resent you. Tell them you have to fit into a new suit, or give them some other specific reason.

- *Cut calories when not at social functions.* During the most tempting festive seasons, trim a moderate amount from your daily breakfast, lunch, and dinner. Every meal, however should be a well-balanced 300 calories or more. Never drop below 300 calories a meal. And never skip meals.

DEALING WITH TV'S SNACK ATTACKS

Watching almost any type of television program is an invitation to overeat. Whether it's football, sitcoms, or cable news, we expose ourselves to that billion-dollar industry that excels at influencing us to enjoy the great taste of some new or old food or drink.

Here is a game plan for dealing with TV's snack attacks:

- A *relish tray* (broccoli, florets of cauliflower, cucumbers, celery, carrots, radishes) with nonfat yogurt as a dip. Drink water flavored with lemon.

- A *fruit salad.* If slicing and dicing is too burdensome, an apple sure can fill you up and provide a great deal of oral gratification. For sweetness, put brown sugar or cinnamon on the apple.

- A *light popcorn* without butter. Sprinkle on Parmesan cheese for extra taste.

- A *frozen banana* for a taste sensation almost like ice cream. *Nonfat frozen yogurt* or *ice milk* would have to be carefully rationed.

- Flavored *coffee* or *tea* to warm your belly. The warmth many times curbs the urge to snack.

- Of the popular things that come in a bag or a box and are so easy to reach into, *pretzels* are less damaging than either corn or potato chips.

HANDLING A VACATION

Summer vacation is supposed to be the spoils of a year of earnest toil. The accumulated stress of nine-to-five workdays are supposed to dissipate in warm sunsets, cool breezes, and the relaxation of having no demands on our time.

Vacations can be—and should be—a stress relief valve. Since many of us fighting a tendency toward fatness overeat in response to stress, relief should assist our calorie control.

But researchers have found the opposite occurring too many times. People try to cram too much into a vacation. And because they want to maximize their enjoyment, instead of disciplining their eating habits, they seek new kinds of taste-bud thrills.

Are you going to bring back excess baggage from your summer vacation? The answer starts with the vacation plan you are probably already making. Here are a few hints.

- Realize that you'll need a couple of days just to slow down from your normal business pace. Don't visit every fun park and museum you can initially.

- Have an activity-oriented plan. Biking, hiking, boating, and mountain climbing are calorie-burning activities that relax and refresh the mind.

- Cool yourself by drinking plenty of water, instead of having high-calorie sodas or ice cream. For a taste sensation, use fruit-based blended drinks or juices.

- Don't mistake the dehydration of sunbathing for activity. Just because you perspire doesn't mean you're burning significant calories.

- Enjoy fine restaurants, but load up on nutrient-dense foods such as salads, vegetables, and broiled fish.

- Set exercise goals for your vacation. Many commercial fitness centers will sell you a pass for a day or week.

- Get into shape for your vacation. Stronger muscles will stamina high.

- Enjoy alcohol sparingly, if at all.

- Read at least one inspiring fitness-related book.

Do not take these suggestions to extremes. Vacations are memory-makers. Their enjoyment is to be relished for years to come.

ADDING AROMAS, COLORS, AND TEXTURES

Most men are attracted to a simple, basic, easy-to-prepare eating plan. As a result, I've tried to keep the Living-Longer-Stronger diet primarily plain vanilla. I also realize, however, that there are men who enjoy experimenting with various seasonings and ingredients that can add some pizzazz to foods which have a reduced level of calories, fat, and salt.

An interesting way to add creativity to basic meals is through foods ingredients that are rich in fragrant *aromas,* vibrant *colors,* and varied *textures,* or A.C.T. A.C.T. is an acronym developed by Graham Kerr, and discussed in his *Creative Choices Cookbook.*

AROMA	COLOR	TEXTURE
Allspice	Beet	Barley
Basil	Bell pepper	Bean sprouts
Chili pepper	Carrot	Capers
Cilantro	Paprika	Radish
Dijon mustard	Parsley	
Garlic	Red cabbage	
Ginger root	Tomato	
Nutmeg		
Tarragon		

A listing of some of these ingredients, as well as a few practical examples, are as follows:

- Freshly ground allspice makes a terrific accent when it is scattered over cooked greens, carrots, or beans.

- Dijon mustard can be used in place of mayonnaise on any sandwich. This great-tasting mustard, which has only 4 calories per teaspoon, combines well with canned tuna.

- Bell peppers come in yellow, red, and green varieties. Their mild, crisp sweetness can add sparkle to any salad. When roasted, they can be used to garnish pasta, fish, and poultry.

- Red cabbage, which is actually purple, may be finely shredded and added raw to vegetables that need color.

- Bean sprouts in several varieties are now available in many supermarkets. They have a fresh, clean taste and texture, which perks up sandwiches of all types.

- Radishes provide unique crispness and bite. Their tart taste and texture will blend with most delicate flavors in salads and sauces.

These examples, as well as many others, are low in calories, but high in aroma, color, or texture. You may use them freely throughout the Living-Longer-Stronger menus.

BACKSLIDING FORWARD

You may have adhered to the Living-Longer-Stronger diet strictly for weeks. Then you wrecked it one day as you walked by a donut shop. Fifteen minutes later you'd wolfed down a half dozen!

You may be progressing nicely with your strength-training routine. An unexpected emergency, however, causes you to miss several workouts.

Now you feel guilty. You broke your diet. You sloughed off on your exercise. You might as well forget the whole program and go back to your old ways.

Stop! Don't let yourself fall into this senseless, destructive trap. Guilt saps your motivation and confidence.

Furthermore, such thinking indicates only a short-term goal. True power revolves around the realization that permanent fat loss is a long-term project that is bound to have ups and downs.

Expect to backslide occasionally. You're only human, right? There is no disgrace in backsliding. The disgrace lies in letting a lapse get you so discouraged that you quit trying. You must move forward.

USE IT OR LOSE IT

If you've lapsed in regard to strength training, the remedy will depend on the length of the lapse. It takes about the same amount of time to lose strength as it takes you to gain it. If you increase the strength of your frontal thigh muscles by 25 percent in six weeks, then it will take you six weeks to lose that strength—given that you do no exercise during that time period.

Thus, for each workout you skip, you must back up a workout in restarting your exercise.

Miss three workouts, then back up three workouts. But take note: Your muscles retain a memory of strength. It's always easier to exercise back to your previous condition than it was originally. Unless it's been many months, you're still ahead of where you started.

Don't lose it. Use it!

EXERCISE-INDUCED HEADACHES

A few people who strength-train may experience what is called an exercise-induced headache. In working with thousands of people over the last 30 years, I've seen it happen perhaps two dozen times. But I've had many phone calls from instructors in fitness centers who have been very concerned for a client who experienced such a headache. Ken Hutchins, author of *Super Slow: The Ultimate Exercise Protocol*, has studied extensively the prevention and treatment of exercise-induced headaches. The guidelines below should help you understand and deal with them.

There are many types of headaches. Some are helped by exercise, others are worsened. A headache may result from caffeine withdrawal, or reduction in dietary calories, as is sometimes experienced by people on the Living-Longer-Stronger program. These types of headaches, as well as tension and migraine headaches, are not the same as exercise-induced headaches. The concern here is for headaches that materialize during strength-training exercise.

Exercise-induced headaches usually occur to inexperienced trainees. Older women seem to be the most susceptible.

Exercise-induced headaches usually occur on machines that involve the hips and thighs. The leg press and leg extension machines are the most prevalent.

Most of the cause of an exercise-induced headache seems to be a weak neck, and an inability to relax the many small muscles that compose the face, neck, and shoulders during the performance on the leg press or leg extension machine.

Here is how to prevent an exercise-induced headache from occurring:

- Stop the exercise immediately if a headache begins to develop during the workout. Do not try to work through the head pain.

- Exit the machine and find a place where you can sit and relax. Do not talk. Keep your eyes closed and remain still for several minutes. If the pain does not vanish, terminate the workout.

- Redefine failure in each exercise. Stop the exercise not when your muscles fail, but at the instant you feel the slightest head pain.

- Make a concentrated effort to relax your face, neck, and shoulders during each lower body exercise. Do not grip excessively with your hands. Do not grit your teeth. Do not hold your breath.

- Continue with your exercise as long as the headache does not return. If the headache returns, stop the workout, relax until it goes away, and go home. Several days later, attempt another workout only if your head pain is nonexistent. If the pain persists for longer than a few days, consult a physician.

- Incorporate the 4-way neck machine (see Chapter 41) into your workouts. Perform the neck exercise first to help relax your neck before doing the other exercises.

- Do the leg exercises last in your workouts.

38

CHECKING YOUR PROGRESS

For the last six weeks you've been losing fat and building muscle. If you've applied yourself according to the instructions, you should definitely see and feel some differences.

To determine your specific results, turn back to Chapter 33 and retake all your body part measurements. When you've finished, you'll want to compare your results to the average expectations.

WINNING BY LOSING

After working with more than 100 men between the ages of 40 and 60 on six-week diet and exercise programs, I calculated their average losses to be as shown to the right.

If you're typical, you should have lost the greatest inches from your waist and thighs: 3½ inches off your waist and 3 inches off your thighs.

AVERAGE INCHES LOST	
Right upper arm	3/8
Left upper arm	3/8
Chest	1¾
Waist	3½
Hips	2
Right thigh	1½
Left thigh	1½
Total inches lost	**11**

How do these inches lost translate to pounds of weight and fat lost?

As I mentioned in previous chapters, most obese men can expect to lose between 3 and 4 pounds of fat per week on the Living-Longer-Stronger program. From the inches diminished above, the men lost an average of 19 pounds of weight and 22 pounds of fat. If you accurately measured your body weight and percent body fat *before* and *after* the six-week program, your improvement should be near these numbers.

Furthermore, if you took whole-body pictures of yourself in a bathing suit six weeks ago, you'll want to retake them again. You should be able to see definite improvement when you compare your *before* and *after* photographs side by side. For valid comparisons, instruct your photo processor to make your *height* in both sets of pictures exactly the same.

WINNING BY BUILDING

Since the average man lost 19 pounds of body weight and 22 pounds of body fat, he must have built 3 pounds of muscle. Building 3 pounds of muscle is typical for the men I worked with on the Living-Longer-Stronger course. That's an average muscle gain of 0.5 pound per week for six weeks.

As I noted earlier, a 0.5 pound per week muscle gain translates to a 5 percent increase in the resistance of each basic strength-training exercise. Thus, over the duration of the six-week program, you'd expect to increase the resistance of your initial six exercises each by approximately 30 percent.

To calculate your strength gain percentage on the basic exercises, look at your workout record for Week 1 and Week 6. For example, for Week 1 on the leg extension, circle in red the first time that you successfully performed 10 repetitions.

LOWERING YOUR CHOLESTEROL

If you follow the Living-Longer-Stronger program, there's a high probability your blood cholesterol level will be reduced. A group of 28 men with whom I worked noted the following average lowering in six weeks:

Total cholesterol	reduced 23 percent
Triglycerides	reduced 27 percent
Total cholesterol/HDL ratio	reduced 9 percent

Then, for Week 6 circle the most recent time you did 10 repetitions. Now subtract initial leg extension resistance from your last leg extension resistance. This number divided by your initial resistance is your percent increase. You can do the same with any exercise as long as the repetitions are identical.

Don't forget, stronger muscles are larger—and larger muscles require more calories at work and rest.

THE NEXT STEP

How do your *after* measurements and results stack up against the averages from my previous studies? Have you reached some of your goals during the last six weeks? Are you presently satisfied or dissatisfied with the way you look and perform?

Part VII will explain how to continue and improve your results, and how to maintain your new leanness and increased strength.

IMPROVING SEXUALITY

Will going through the Living-Longer-Stronger program, besides the obvious loss of fat and gain of muscle, improve your sex life?

Although I haven't done any research in this area, others have. Generally research reveals that as a man goes from fatness to fitness, and his overall health improves, so does his interest in sex.

It is true that men in their 40s and beyond—compared to men in their 20s—are more likely to suffer from obesity, high blood pressure, cholesterol buildup, low back pain, and knee problems, all of which can negatively affect their sexual behavior. The Living-Longer-Stronger program can successfully treat each of these conditions.

One study, for example, found that the heart isn't the only organ affected by a buildup of cholesterol. Cholesterol can clog the blood vessels in and around the penis, making erections weak and difficult to sustain.

I know for sure that proper dieting and proper exercising can reverse the buildup of cholesterol. Furthermore, strength training boosts blood flow and increases circulation—all of which makes for stronger erections.

Other studies have found that strength training can actually increase testosterone levels, which piques sexual interest. One group of men between the ages of 40 and 80 registered a strong correlation between vigorous physical conditioning and sexual frequency and pleasure.

William Masters and Virginia Johnson, the famed sex researchers, recognized over 30 years ago that post-menopausal women displayed greater sexual interest than their partners. These women often wished their men could keep up with their revived sexual energy.

I believe now, with *Living Longer Stronger*, men can regain and even increase their sexual capacity. If we live longer stronger, and we certainly can, then we can also love longer stronger.

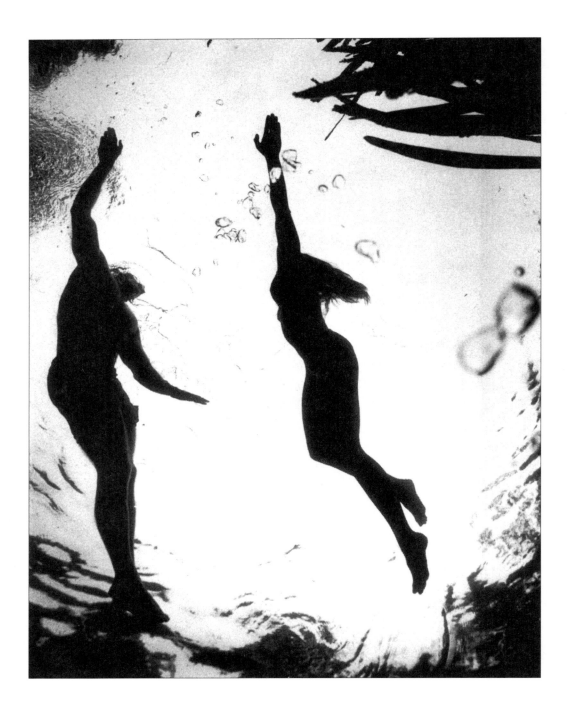

VII.
REJUVENATING
YOUR
LIFE

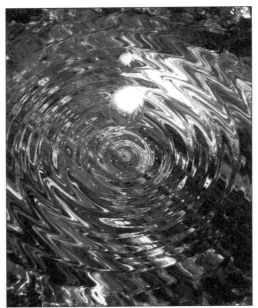

Losing fat and building muscle produce a ripple effect on other aspects of your life. For example, they can exert confidence and control in the midst of confusion and complexity.

39
IMPROVING YOUR RESULTS

Maybe you lost 15, 20, or even 25 pounds of fat on the six-week course, but you've still got more pounds and inches to lose. It took you longer than six weeks to put it on—try 20 years—and it's going to take a little more time to get it off.

You probably have to weigh well over 250 pounds to lose 35 pounds of fat or more in six weeks. Yes, Larry Freedman, whom you met in Chapter 32, removed 52¾ pounds. But Larry weighed 306 pounds when he started, and he was an exceptional individual. So, if you weigh less than 250 pounds and have more than 30 pounds of fat to eliminate, there's a high probability that it's going to require longer than six weeks. If you're in this category, here's what to do.

MAKE ANOTHER COMMITMENT

Decide now that you want to continue. You've already taken some major steps toward removing your excess body fat. You've made significant progress by sticking with the plan for six weeks. Make a commitment for another six weeks, or less, if you believe you can reach your goal sooner.

Some men require three or four times, 18 to 24 weeks, before they reach their satisfaction level. Simply turn the week-by-week dieting, exercising, and other practices into week-by-week steps which move you closer and closer to your goal.

TAKE A WEEK OFF

You may think I'm contradicting myself if I tell you to take a week off after I just asked you to make a commitment to further dieting and exercising. Most of the men who continued with the plan felt that a week off renewed their enthusiasm.

Be careful not to gorge yourself with food. You probably would have difficulty doing so even if you tried. Simply eat approximately 500 more calories per day than you were eating during Weeks 5 and 6—or approximately 1,800 calories a day. Keep drinking your water: 1⅝ gallons a day.

After a week off you'll be amazed at how eager you are to repeat the six-week course.

REPEAT THE DIET

Six weeks ago, in two-week phases, you gradually descreased your calories from 1,500 to 1,400 to 1,300 per day. Now that you've added a few pounds of muscle to your body, you should be able to progress through the same descending-calorie plan with similar results.

Furthermore, this time around you'll be more familiar with the menus and foods. You'll be able to gauge serving sizes without actually weighing and measuring. The entire process will be easier. Just be sure your daily calories remain at the appropriate level.

You may be wondering why this down-up-down plan is recommended in preference to sticking to the same number of calories each day, week, and month. The down-up-down method is effective for three reasons:

- Such a diet supplies you with needed variety.

- A certain irregularity exists which seems to benefit your body's fat-burning process.

- When your calories go up, so does your energy level. Such an increase in energy level may be just the motivation you need to train harder and thus stimulate additional muscle growth.

You can continue this down-up-down eating plan for as long as six months, or until you attain your fat-loss goal.

CONTINUE YOUR STRENGTH TRAINING

During the last two weeks of the six-week program, you did one set of ten exercises during each of your training sessions. You should continue with this routine of ten exercises three times per week until you lose your excess fat. Don't do less or more than ten exercises.

Your strength-training goal is to double your strength in all your basic exercises. If you did 100 pounds for 10 repetitions on the leg extension machine when you started, for example, then your goal is to perform 200 pounds for 10 repetitions. Many men can reach that goal within four to six months on all their basic exercises.

Once this goal is reached, you should modify your routine by adding some different exercises to your workout. The next two chapters discuss how this is accomplished.

Your other practices—such as water drinking, walking, and extra sleeping—should remain unchanged from Weeks 5 and 6.

CONCENTRATE ONE DAY AT A TIME

Patience is truly a virtue when it comes to losing those last few pounds of fat.

Hang in there. Those fat cells can shrink. Your dream, if it is realistic, can be accomplished. It does take time, however.

Be patient. Stick to the plan in this book. Take it one day at a time.

Make intelligent action your ally.

40
MAINTENANCE GUIDELINES

Once you become satisfied with the condition of your body—whether it takes six weeks, twelve weeks, or more—your next task is to maintain that status. Doing so requires certain adjustments to the guidelines and practices that you've been applying for the last several months.

Study carefully the following adjustments.

ADHERE TO A CARBOHYDRATE-RICH, MODERATE-CALORIE EATING PLAN

Your eating plan is still carbohydrate-rich, but you do not need to decrease the calories. Your calories are now raised to a moderate level. Instead of eating from 1,300 to 1,500 calories a day, you'll be consuming from 1,800 to 2,400 calories per day. Maybe you can even eat more after your new body weight has stabilized.

There is no simple way to determine in advance how many calories you will need to maintain your new body weight. Trial-and-error experimentation will make the level obvious, however.

You should probably begin with 1,800 calories per day and see what happens after a week. If your body weight keeps going down, raise the calories to 1,900 or 2,000, depending on how much weight you lost during the last week. Soon, you should reach a level where your body weight stabilizes. That level is your daily calorie requirement.

Always keep your calories rich in carbohydrates. The 60:20:20 ratio of carbohydrates, proteins, and fats is not only ideal for losing fat, but it is also appropriate for maintenance. Fruits, vegetables, breads, and cereals are your primary sources of carbohydrates. On your maintenance eating plan, strive each day to consume six servings of fruits and vegetables and six servings of breads and cereals. Doing so will usually allow your other foods—meats and dairy products—to fall into correct ratio naturally. Also, reread Chapter 19 for suggestions on breakfast, lunch, and dinner.

EAT SMALLER MEALS MORE FREQUENTLY

You've been limiting your five meals per day to 500 calories or less. To maintain your body weight, set the limit per meal to 600 calories or less. A 600-calorie meal will still keep your insulin responses small. Furthermore, 600-calorie meals are something you can easily adapt to—at least, most of the time.

What happens when you occasionally eat more than 600 calories at one time? Don't panic. Simply understand that you will sometimes backslide. Anticipate, plan, and get back on track.

DRINK 128 OUNCES OF COLD WATER EACH DAY

I hope by now you've seen and felt the benefits of drinking plenty of cold water each day. Make it a permanent part of your new lifestyle to consume at least 128 ounces or one gallon of water each day, and more when you can.

PERFORM STRENGTH TRAINING TWO TIMES PER WEEK

You never outgrow your need for larger, stronger muscles. As you age, larger and stronger muscles become more and more important. In fact, that's the theme of this entire book. Bigger muscles improve performance, add shape, stabilize joints, burn more calories, and consequently allow you to live longer stronger.

There are two primary differences between your maintenance routines and your past workouts. First, during maintenance you can introduce more variety to your routine by adding some new exercises while removing some old ones. Chapter 41 details how this is done. Second, with maintenance, you can reduce your frequency of exercise from three to two times per week. Remember, as your muscles get stronger, you actually need less total exercise.

WALK AFTER YOUR EVENING MEAL

Walking on a full stomach is a great way to relax and burn extra calories. Although you may not feel it's necessary to do so every day of the week, you should still take advantage of this effect frequently during your maintenance plan.

Sleep an Extra Hour Each Night

Extra sleep is like extra water: you didn't know what you were missing until you tried it. It will be to your advantage to maintain your new sleeping schedule every night you can.

Practice Other Fat-Loss Facts

You may apply the fat-loss facts from Chapter 30 anytime they are needed during your maintenance program. With an understanding of these facts, your arsenal should remain well stocked.

Avoid Overstress

Some medical authorities believe that overstress is the real culprit behind obesity, high blood pressure, heart disease, the divorce rate, and just about everything else that plagues today's aging businessman. Certainly, too much stress can seriously limit your body's ability to lose fat. And too much stress can ruin your maintenance plan and cause a return to your old ways of coping. Don't let this happen to you.

Stay calm and stay in control.

41
NEW STRENGTH-TRAINING ROUTINES

Your maintenance strength-training routines bring into action all the exercises that were listed in Chapter 18. So far, your exercise routines have been basic. You'll now get a chance to add some variety to your workouts.

Variety in exercise is good to a degree. But many men involved with strength training carry variety too far. They perform too many different exercises and never really master the mechanics of the basic movements.

In Chapter 18, I noted that there were more than 500 strength-training movements that you could perform with machines, barbells, and dumbbells. From this list, however, I focused on the best 30 exercises, which were broken into 15 performed with machines and 15 done with barbells and dumbbells.

During Weeks 1 through 6, you utilized a routine that included ten machine exercises or ten barbell and dumbbell exercises. Now, the unused five machine exercises and five barbell-dumbbell exercises will be incorporated into the new workouts.

There are four maintenance routines involving machines and another four applying to barbells and dumbbells. Each routine still has only 10 exercises. The recommended way to use the routines is as follows:

- Perform Maintenance Routine 1 three times a week for two weeks.

- Perform Maintenance Routine 2 three times a week for the next two weeks.

- Alternate between Routine 1 and Routine 2 for two more weeks. In other words, one week do Routine 1 on Monday and Friday, and Routine 2 on Wednesday. The next week perform Routine 2 twice and Routine 1 once.

Thus in six weeks, you will have mastered all 15 basic exercises. This is a good time to add a little more variety with Routine 3, which emphasizes your upper arms, and Routine 4, which specializes on your chest. Here's the suggested way to employ these new routines:

- Apply Maintenance Routine 3 or Maintenance Routine 4 three times a week for two weeks.

- Make sure you get plenty of rest on your non-training days.

- Go back to Maintenance Routine 1 and 2 and alternate between them for two weeks to a month.

- Try Routine 3 or 4 for another two weeks.

- Keep this revolving pattern in your exercise program for as long as you are satisfied with your results.

- Reduce your workouts from three times per week to two times per week, as soon as you reach a training plateau.

- Continue to train twice a week, following the same two-week patterns, from here on.

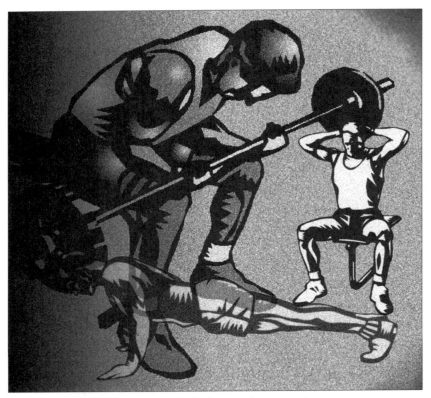

Remember to stress good form on all the exercises in your maintenance workouts.

MACHINE ROUTINES

MAINTENANCE ROUTINE 1

1. Leg Extension or Leg Curl
2. Leg Press
3. Standing Calf Raise*
4. Lateral Raise
5. Pullover
6. Bench Press
7. Behind Neck Pulldown*
8. Triceps Extension
9. Biceps Curl
10. 4-Way Neck*

* Indicates new exercise

MAINTENANCE ROUTINE 2

1. Leg Curl
2. Leg Extension
3. Standing Calf Raise
4. 10° Chest*
5. Behind Neck Pulldown
6. Bench Press
7. Biceps Curl
8. Lower Back
9. Abdominal
10. Rotary Torso*

* Indicates new exercise

MAINTENANCE ROUTINE 3 ARM EMPHASIS

1. Leg Curl
2. Leg Extension
3. Leg Press
4. Lateral Raise
5. Pullover
6. Triceps Extension
7. Bench Press
8. Biceps Curl
9. Behind Neck Pulldown
10. Abdominal or Lower Back

Note: The exercises inside the brackets should be performed with minimum rest between them.

MAINTENANCE ROUTINE 4 CHEST EMPHASIS

1. Leg Curl
2. Leg Extension
3. Standing Calf Raise
4. 10° Chest
5. Bench Press
6. Push-Up on Floor
7. Behind Neck Pulldown
8. Triceps Extension
9. Rotary Torso
10. 4-Way Neck

Note: The exercises inside the brackets should be performed with minimum rest between them.

DESCRIPTIONS OF NEW MACHINE EXERCISES

Standing Calf Raise Machine

Muscles worked: This is the standard exercise for building your gastrocnemius, or back calf, muscles. It can be performed on a variety of machines.

Starting position: Face the machine and bend your knees enough so that you can position your shoulders beneath the yoke of the machine. Stand and place your feet shoulder-width apart on the toe block or step, with only your toes and the balls of your feet in contact with the block. Straighten your knees and keep them locked throughout the exercise. Sag your heels as far below the level of your toes as comfortably possible. Keep your feet pointed straight ahead.

Exercise performance: Raise your heels smoothly in 4 seconds and try to stand on your tiptoes. Do not bend your knees. Pause briefly in the highest position. Lower slowly to the bottom and stretch. Repeat for maximum repetitions.

Training tips: Many bodybuilders are convinced that turning their toes in during calf raises works more of the lateral head of the gastrocnemius. Likewise, turning the toes out involves more of the medial head. Such techniques, however, are unfounded since the origin and insertion points of the gastrocnemius are not altered by foot placement.

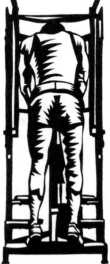

Contracted position

Behind Neck Pulldown Machine

Mid-range position

Muscles worked: The pulldown involves your biceps and latissimus dorsi muscles.

Starting position: There are a variety of pulldown machines and bars that are available. The best choice is a bar that allows a parallel grip with your hands approximately 24 inches apart. If a parallel-grip bar is not available, use an underhand grip. Stabilize yourself under the bar. Grasp the overhead bar.

Exercise performance: Pull the bar smoothly behind your neck. Pause. Return slowly to the stretched position. Repeat for 8 to 12 repetitions.

Training tips: Avoid spacing your hands farther apart than 24 inches. A wide grip limits your range of movement and makes the exercise less productive.

4-Way Neck Machine

Muscles worked: There are over a dozen small and medium-sized muscles that make up your neck's mass. Collectively they are called the neck extensor group and neck flexor group. These muscle groups are weak and underdeveloped in most men in their second middle age.

Starting position: For the first several months, you should only do the back extension part of the 4-way neck machine. Adjust the seat so that while you are seated erect your throat is on the same level as the axis of rotation of the movement arm. Enter the machine with the back of your head against the center of the pad. Stabilize your torso by grasping the handles lightly.

Exercise performance: Push the head pad upward while straightening your spine and raising your chest. Continue pushing the pad backward while moving your shoulders forward. Extend your head as far back as comfortably possible. Pause. Return slowly to the starting position. Repeat for 8 to 12 repetitions.

Training tips: Be alert and focused on this machine, especially since your neck and cervical spine are vulnerable. Do not jerk on any repetition. After you've doubled your strength on the back extension exercise, you may add the front flexion and lateral contractions to your workouts.

Contracted position

10° Chest Machine

Muscles worked: The 10° chest machine isolates the pectoralis major muscles without involving your triceps.

Starting position: Lie on your back with your head higher than your hips. Your head should be almost touching the upholstery at the top of the bench. Place your upper arms under the roller pads. The pads should be in the crooks of your elbows.

Exercise performance: Move your arms in a rotary fashion until the roller pads touch over your chest. Pause. Lower slowly to the starting position. Repeat for maximum repetitions.

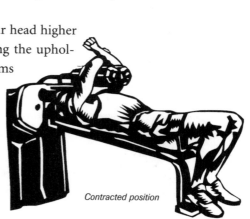

Contracted position

Training tips: In the stretched position, when viewed from the side, it is important to keep your hands, elbows, and shoulders in line with one another. This directs the resistance on your chest muscles.

Rotary Torso Machine

Muscles worked: This machine zeros in on the external and internal obliques muscles, which lie on both sides of your waist.

Starting position: Straddle the seat. Make sure it is locked into the extreme right or left position. Anchor your lower body by crossing your ankles. Position your head and spinal column directly above the movement arm's pivot point. Fasten the belt across your thighs. Place your upper arms securely over the angled roller pads behind your back. Your elbows should be as close together as comfortably possible.

Exercise performance: Allow the back pressure of the movement arm to rotate your torso in one direction for a moderate stretch. Rotate smoothly to the opposite side. Pause. Return slowly to stretched position. Repeat for maximum repetitions. Adjust the seat to the opposite side and work your other side.

Training tips: For better isolation, pretend that your arms and torso are fused together, so that you cannot move your arms without moving your torso. As you twist, you'll feel the action more in your waist.

Starting position

Push-Up on Floor

Muscles worked: The push-up is performed third in the chest cycle of Maintenance Routine 4. It works your triceps, deltoids, and pectoral muscles.

Starting position: Lie face down on the floor with your hands under your shoulders. Get on your toes and stiffen your knees, hips, and torso.

Exercise performance: Straighten your arms and lift your body. Bend your elbows and lower your chest to barely touch the floor. Repeat for maximum repetitions.

Training tips: The push-up will be extremely difficult to do immediately after the other two chest exercises. You may have to cheat in pushing

Top position

up by using your knees and hips. If so, concentrate more on the lowering phase of the movement. Force out as many slow, lowering repetitions as you can.

FORCED REPETITIONS

When you reach momentary muscular failure on the positive portion of an exercise, you usually terminate the set. But if your partner helps you by lifting up on the bar or movement arm, you can successfully lower the resistance negatively for several more repetitions. Such assistance is called *forced repetitions*.

Forced repetitions allow you to exhaust your negative strength, as well as positive strength on a given exercise. Initially, if you've never tried forced repetitions, they will produce very good results. This is probably due to the negative exhaustion factor.

Most trainees, however, carry a good thing too far. They start applying forced repetitions during each set of every workout, which probably means they are overtraining. Or, in their haste to get to the forced repetition, they fail to work to muscular exhaustion on the initial positive movements, which usually leads to a gradual reduction in the intensity of exercise.

If you know that you are going to be subjected to forced repetitions at the end of a normal set, you usually fail to produce a complete effort during the normal repetitions. You will stop one or two movements short of an all-out effort in preparation for an optimum display of strength during the following forced repetitions.

In either situation, it soon becomes very difficult to record briefly and accurately on a workout card what has been accomplished.

The full benefit of forced repetitions occurs when your training partner only *occasionally* applies this technique, perhaps once every two weeks. Even then, you should not be aware that you are going to do forced repetitions until you have completed your last possible normal repetition. Do not underestimate the element of surprise in the application of forced repetitions.

BARBELL-DUMBBELL ROUTINES

MAINTENANCE ROUTINE 1

1. Squat with Barbell
2. Pullover with Dumbbell
3. Overhead Press with Barbell*
4. Prone Back Raise
5. Biceps Curl with Barbell
6. Triceps Extension with Dumbbell
7. Lateral Raise with Dumbbells
8. Bench Press with Barbell
9. Trunk Curl
10. Neck Extension Against Hand Resistance*

* Indicates new exercise

MAINTENANCE ROUTINE 2

1. Stiff-Legged Deadlift with Barbell
2. One-Legged Calf Raise with Dumbbell
3. Negative Chin-Up*
4. Negative Dip*
5. Lateral Raise with Dumbbells
6. Bench Press with Barbell
7. Biceps Curl with Barbell
8. Overhead Press with Barbell
9. Wrist Curl with Barbell*
10. Trunk Curl

* Indicates new exercise

MAINTENANCE ROUTINE 3 ARM EMPHASIS

1. Squat with Barbell
2. Prone Back Raise
3. Lateral Raise with Dumbbells
4. Pullover with Dumbbell
5. Triceps Extension with Dumbbell
6. Negative Dip
7. Biceps Curl with Barbell
8. Negative Chin-Up
9. Wrist Curl with Barbell
10. Trunk Curl

Note: The exercises inside the brackets should be performed with minimum rest between them.

MAINTENANCE ROUTINE 4 CHEST EMPHASIS

1. Squat with Barbell
2. One-Legged Calf Raise with Dumbbell
3. Stiff-Legged Deadlift with Barbell
4. Bench Press with Barbell
5. Negative Dip
6. Push-Up on Floor
7. Negative Chin-Up
8. Triceps Extension with Dumbbell
9. Prone Back Raise
10. Neck Extension Against Hand Resistance

Note: The exercises inside the brackets should be performed with minimum rest between them.

DESCRIPTIONS OF NEW BARBELL-DUMBBELL EXERCISES

Overhead Press with Barbell

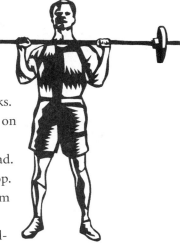

Starting position

Muscles worked: This exercise involves your deltoids and triceps.

Starting position: Load the barbell on the squat racks. Grasp the barbell with a palms-up grip and stand erect. Position it on your shoulders with your hands shoulder-width apart.

Exercise performance: Press the barbell smoothly overhead. Do not lock out your elbows. Keep a slight bend in them at the top. Lower the barbell slowly to your shoulders. Repeat for maximum repetitions.

Training tips: Do not bounce the barbell off your shoulders. Do not arch your back excessively during the pressing.

Neck Extension Against Hand Resistance

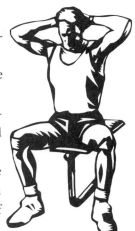

Starting position

Muscles worked: Over a dozen small and medium-sized neck muscles are stressed in this exercise.

Starting position: Interlace your fingers and place them on the back of your head. Position your chin on your chest.

Exercise performance: Push your head back and resist the movement with your hands and arms. Then pull forward with your arms and resist with your neck muscles. Repeat for 8 to 12 repetitions.

Training tips: Ease into this exercise gradually. Keep the resistance steady. After you've significantly strengthened the back of your neck, you can add a similar movement with hand resistance for the front and sides of your neck.

Negative Chin-Up

Muscles worked: Remember, the negative part of the exercise is the lowering phase. So on a negative chin-up, the emphasis is on moving downward very slowly. Properly performed, this exercise is one of the most productive for your biceps and latissimus dorsi.

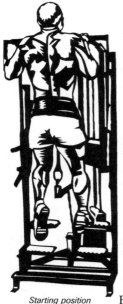

Starting position

Starting position: You do not use the standard 4 seconds up and 4 seconds down in this exercise. Instead, you do the positive work with your legs and the negative work with your upper body. Place a chair or bench under a chinning bar. Climb onto the chair and get into the top position with your chin over the bar. Use an underhand grip and space your hands shoulder-width apart.

Exercise performance: Remove your feet from the chair and lower your body slowly in 10 seconds. Make sure you come all the way down to a dead hang. Quickly climb back to the top position with your chin over the bar. Repeat the slow lowering for maximum repetitions.

Training tips: Your strength should increase rapidly on the negative chin-up. Soon you'll be able to strap or hang additional weight around your hips. Here are the guidelines to follow:

During your first several negative repetitions, you should take 10 seconds to lower your body. If you had to, you could stop the downward movement. But don't. Continue to lower in 10 seconds. After five or six repetitions, if the weight is selected correctly, you should be able to control the downward movement, but *not* stop it. When you can no longer control your negative repetition, stop. In other words, the entire lowering portion will be completed in 2 or 3 seconds, in spite of your best efforts to reduce the speed. When you can do ten or more repetitions in good form, add more weight around your hips.

Mid-range position

Negative Dip

Muscles worked: Negative dips involve your pushing muscles: triceps, deltoids, and pectoralis majors.

Starting position: You may require extra resistance added to your body weight for maximum results from negative dips. Place a sturdy chair or bench between a set of parallel bars. Climb into the top position and straighten your arms. Remove your feet from the chair and stabilize your body.

Exercise performance: Bend your arms and lower your body smoothly in 10 seconds. Stretch comfortably in the bottom position. Climb back to the starting position and straighten your arms. Repeat the slow lowering for maximum repetitions.

Training tips: Keep the time between negative repetitions as brief as possible. Quickly climb back to the top position. Do not take longer than 3 seconds on the climb. In fact, 2 seconds is even better. Taking a longer time between negative repetitions allows your involved muscles a chance to recover partially.

Wrist Curl with Barbell

Muscles worked: This exercise stresses the flexor muscles of your forearms.

Starting position: Grasp a barbell with a palms-up grip. Rest your forearms on your thighs and the backs of your hands against your knees, and be seated. Lean forward until the angle between your upper arms and forearms is less than 90 degrees. This position allows you to isolate your forearms more completely.

Exercise performance: Curl the barbell smoothly and contract your forearm muscles. Pause briefly. Lower the barbell slowly. Repeat for maximum repetitions.

Training tips: Since this is such a short range of motion, it's easy to cheat on this exercise. Resist that temptation. Keep your repetitions slow and strict, and your forearms will respond rapidly.

Contracted position

MAKING PROGRESS

It's important still to keep accurate records of all your maintenance routines. The blank chart from Chapter 36 may be used for any maintenance routine, or for any future workout that you may design yourself. In fact, after six months of strength training under your belt, you and your partner should be able to add some new twists to your workouts. One of my previous books, *100 High-Intensity Ways to Improve Your Bodybuilding*, can provide some additional help as well.

42

OVERLEARNING:
THE FORGOTTEN SECRET

I rarely use the word *secret* in my writings. I avoid it because it's associated with tabloid headlines that promote gimmicks and unscientific findings.

The subject of this chapter, however, is an exception. Discovering it was like I had suddenly found a treasure box that had been misplaced and forgotten for many years.

Opening that box, in my mind, revealed a real secret. It's a secret, however, that needs to be shared with everyone who has lost fat and regained it. For when you understand this concept you'll be able to maintain your fat loss permanently.

REDISCOVERING THE SECRET

The secret I'm talking about was revealed to me in the summer of 1992. I was browsing in the Alachua County Library when a title caught my eye: *Keeping It Off: Winning at Weight Loss* by Drs. Robert H. Colvin and Susan C. Olson. Thumbing through this book made me aware of this forgotten secret—*overlearning*.

Overlearning means any practice after a certain level of achievement. In scientific journals, the criterion of success is usually one perfect trial. A trial, for example, may consist of learning ten nonsense syllables or making a foul shot in basketball. Researchers have studied the effects of practice beyond the point when criterion learning has occurred and have come to the same conclusion: overlearning results in better retention of the material learned than regular learning.

No amount of practice seems enough for the serious-minded athlete. Larry Bird, the now-retired all-pro basketball superstar, estimates that he shot the ball at the basket not thousands of times, not hundreds of thousands of times—but millions of times! Overlearning is one reason why Bird is such a superb shooter.

Is it any wonder that even after years of no practice, former college athletes can still demonstrate a high degree of proficiency in their areas of specialty? Of course, the average individual does not desire and perhaps lacks the ability to attain such a high level of skill. Although his time involvement will be considerably less than that of the college or professional athlete, it should be remembered that more practice will increase the potential for later-in-life skills.

What do successful athletes have in common with successful dieters? The answer is *overlearning*.

Reading *Keeping It Off* made me aware of the connection. Yes, I had studied about it years ago in graduate school at Florida State University, but the information failed to stick with me. I certainly didn't overlearn it.

OVERLEARNING AND FAT LOSS

Overlearning, as it relates to fat loss, means the practicing of certain behaviors again and again until they are so ingrained that almost nothing can disturb them. Overlearning produces automatic actions. Without thinking, you demonstrate the correct behavior. The more times you experience the desired response, the better you get and the more lasting is the pattern.

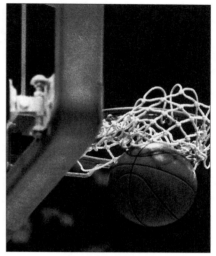

Practice makes perfect only if the practice is perfect. Perfect practice requires overlearning of the basics. Overlearning of the basics is essential for success in basketball, tennis, golf, and other sports—as well as fat loss.

Throughout their book, Drs. Colvin and Olsen interview dieters who have lost from 20 to 275 pounds, the average being 53.2 pounds, and who have kept the weight off for an average of six years. After studying all the interviews, I came to the conclusion that the main ingredient for success is overlearning. All of the subjects followed a predictable pattern to permanent weight loss that they kept repeating daily, weekly, and monthly.

Of the 98 people who successfully finished the original Nautilus Diet plan at the Gainesville Health & Fitness Center, Gainesville, Florida, in 1985, as well as thousands more who have completed similar courses since then, the ones who have kept their lost fat off have done so because of overlearning. The salient guidelines—such as eat smaller meals more frequently, drink at least one gallon of water each day, perform strength training three times per week, and sleep an extra hour each night—have been internalized.

In spite of financial difficulties, lawsuits, divorce, life-threatening illnesses, serious accidents, and the deaths of family and friends, they have not regained their lost fat. It is not because their lost weight is more important than such tragedies—

far from it—but the habits acquired through practice are so deeply established that they persist even when stressful events come to the forefront.

There's an old Texas saying that gets it across: "Dance with the one who brung ya!" In other words, the guidelines and behaviors that got your fat off are the same ones to apply to keep it off. The entire process is much easier if the guidelines are overlearned.

100 DAYS!

How long does it take for overlearning to occur? Behavioral psychologists say that it takes 21 days to establish a pattern and 100 days to make it automatic.

I've observed similar time spans among my group participants. The Living-Longer-Stronger program gets easier for most men after three weeks. If they stick with the discipline for three months, their daily behaviors adapt and become almost automatic. These men then have a high probability of keeping their lost fat off permanently.

You might say, therefore, that overlearning in eating and exercising requires 100 days. But is that truly overlearning? With some men, yes. With others, no. My experience in working with thousands of men shows that 200 days of practice is better than 100. Within reason, more is better.

PRACTICE AND MORE PRACTICE

Practice, practice, and more practice of proper eating and exercising is the key to losing fat. More importantly, because you are building a strong shield against the temptation to return to your old ways of coping, overpractice is the key to keeping off your lost fat permanently.

Make the forgotten secret of overlearning work for you.

43
LIVING LONGER STRONGER

I'm sure most of you looked at comic books when you were growing up. On the back cover of almost every issue during the 1940s was a Charles Atlas advertisement.

THE 97-POUND WEAKLING

Remember how the pitch opened? There's Mac, a puny teenager—probably a sophomore in high school—enjoying a day at the beach with his girlfriend. Along comes a big bully, who runs by and kicks sand in the kids' faces. Mac hollers at the bully and jumps to his feet partly thinking the huge guy will keep on running.

Instead, the bully stops, walks back, grabs Mac by the arm, looks him in the eye, and says: "I'd smash your face . . . only you're so skinny you might dry up and blow away."

As Mac cowers in his tracks, the bully confidently strides off. The girl quickly gets up, shakes her head at Mac, and says, "Oh don't let it bother you, little boy!" Then, she admiringly follows the big guy to his part of the beach. Mac is humiliated and hurries away.

The scene shifts. That night, Mac is reading in his room when he notices the Charles Atlas ad. He tears out the coupon and mails it in.

FROM A MOUSE TO A HE-MAN

The scene changes again. Mac has received the Atlas bodybuilding course and has been secretly training at home for several months. His once puny body has been transformed into mounds of rock-hard muscles. As he flexes his arms in the mirror at home, he thinks to himself: "With these muscles, that bully won't shove me around again!"

The next day, Mac goes back to the beach. Soon he sees the bully showing off in front of a crowd, which includes his old girlfriend. Fearlessly, Mac strides up, dukes out his rival, wins back his girlfriend, and draws sexy stares from the other girls.

THE JOY OF GETTING EVEN

The Charles Atlas ad had great power. I ordered the course when I was a teenager, and so did many of you. In fact, the same ad ran virtually unchanged in comic books for 60 years.

The amazing appeal of the ad for many of us turned out to be something different from what was suspected at first. Was Mac beefing up to prove his love for the girl? Hardly. In fact, the last scene at the beach suggests that Mac soon moves on to greener pastures. Mac's primary motivation was revenge, or the joy of getting even. By getting even, Mac progressed from being controlled to being in control.

It was difficult being a teenager, wasn't it? We weren't in control very much of the time. And what we could control, we enjoyed. That's why bigger, stronger muscles helped. So did success in sports. Both assisted us in competition. Both helped us be in control.

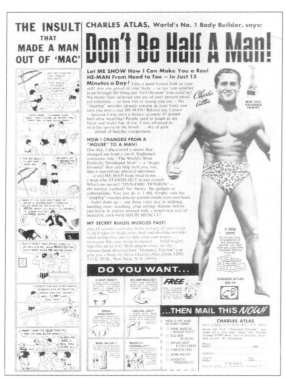

Stronger muscles were the key to Charles Atlas's success. Stronger muscles are also the key to living longer.

MAC IN HIS SECOND MIDDLE AGE

The Living-Longer-Stronger program today is like the Charles Atlas ad of yesterday. Mac, however, is no longer a teenager. He's going on 50. His once-proud muscles have atrophied, his belly has ballooned, his health has eroded, and sand is being kicked in his face once again.

It's time for Mac to get motivated and get back in control. As he did some 35 years ago, he must start with the basics: *his muscles!*

Bigger, stronger muscles will put Mac in control again. His advantage today is that the Living-Longer-Stronger program is light-years ahead of the Charles Atlas course.

BACK IN CONTROL

If you've applied the Living-Longer-Stronger plan for several months, then you know what I'm talking about. First, you rebuild your muscle and reduce your fat. Second, you rethink, rework, and relearn the basics. Third, you recharge your life.

Living Longer Stronger puts you in control of your own destiny.

PROPER STRENGTH TRAINING

At the center of the Living-Longer-Stronger program is strength training. Proper strength training, as you have experienced it throughout this course, provides the following benefits:

- Enlarged muscular size and strength

- Enhanced joint flexibility

- Improved cardiovascular endurance or aerobic capacity

- Increased bone density

- Elevated basal metabolic rate

- Decreased body fat

Furthermore, proper strength training indirectly supplies additional advantages:

- Controlled blood-sugar level

- Improved cholesterol/HDL ratio

- Lowered blood pressure

- Regulated internal temperature

- Reduced risk of injury

You can see why the biomarkers described in Chapter 1 made international headlines when the facts about them were published in 1991. The benefits of strength training will continue to receive featured billing in your own life as you progress in your Living-Longer-Stronger program.

LIVING-LONGER-STRONGER RULES

Let's briefly summarize the most important principles that you've utilized throughout this book and must apply for lifelong success.

- Muscles are the engines of your body. Strengthen your engines, and you'll live longer.

- Strength training applies meaningful resistance to work your targeted muscles to the point of momentary muscular failure.

- Proper strength training not only enlarges your skeletal muscles, but enhances your joint flexibility and increases your cardiovascular endurance.

- The key to long-term progress in strength training is to exercise *harder* and *briefer.* Doing so is an indication that you are also training *smarter.*

- The ideal fat-loss eating plan for men contains from 1,500 to 1,300 calories per day, which are broken down as follows: carbohydrates, 60 percent; fats, 20 percent; and proteins, 20 percent.

- Eating smaller meals more often, with none of the meals exceeding 600 calories, is an important aspect of efficient fat loss.

- Drinking at least a gallon of cold water each day facilitates fat reduction and many other body functions.

- Too much stress in your life limits your ability to lose fat and build muscle.

- Maintenance studies reveal that it takes 21 days to establish a pattern and 100 days to make it automatic.

- The more you overlearn the most important principles, the higher the probability is that your changes are permanent.

Remember, the Living-Longer-Stronger principles have to be ongoing. You must be persistent with them. Interruptions in your exercising and eating patterns will cause your strength and leanness to deteriorate. Your body reacts positively when you exercise, eat, and recover properly. It reacts negatively when you don't. It's just that *simple.*

PARTING THOUGHTS

The days that make up your second middle age slip away quickly. Many men never come close to reaching their revitalization capacity. Don't let this happen to you.

Decide now that you're going to be consistent with your strength training, proactive eating, and factual practicing. Take advantage of each day, each week, and each month—and enjoy

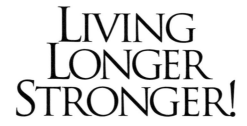

BIBLIOGRAPHY

"Are You Eating Right?" *Consumer Reports* 58:644–655, October 1992.

Ballor, Douglas L. "Set Your Pace: Do You Know the Secret to Burning Body Fat?" *Shape* 9:63–64, December, 1989.

Barrett, Stephen, and Jarvis, William T. *The Health Robbers.* Buffalo, New York: Prometheus Books, 1993.

Bronte, Lydia. *The Longevity Factor.* New York: Harper-Collins, 1993.

Chui, Edward. "The Effect of Systematic Weight Training on Athletic Power," *Research Quarterly* 21:188–194, 1950.

Colvin, Robert A., and Olson, Susan C. *Keeping It Off: Winning at Weight Loss.* New York: Simon & Schuster, 1985.

Cooper, Kenneth A. *Aerobics.* New York: Bantam Books, 1968.

Cornacchia, Harold J., and Barrett, Stephen. *Consumer Health: A Guide to Intelligent Decisions.* St. Louis: Mosby, 1993.

Darden, Ellington. *Soft Steps to a Hard Body.* Dallas: Taylor Publishing Co., 1993.

_____. *High-Intensity Strength Training.* New York: Perigee, 1992.

_____. *32 Days to a 32-Inch Waist.* Dallas: Taylor Publishing Co., 1990.

_____. *The Nautilus Book.* Chicago: Contemporary Books, 1990.

_____. *100 High-Intensity Ways to Improve Your Bodybuilding.* New York: Perigee, 1989.

_____. *The Nautilus Diet.* Boston: Little, Brown and Co., 1987.

Davis, J. Mark et al. "Weight Control and Calorie Expenditure: Thermogenesis Effects of Pre-Prandial and Post-Prandial Exercise," *Addictive Behaviors* 14:347–351, 1989.

DeLorme, Thomas L., and Watkins, Arthur L. *Progressive Resistance Exercise.* New York: Appleton-Century-Crofts, Inc., 1951.

Douglas, Ben H. *AgeLess.* Brandon, MS: QRP Books, 1990.

Evans, William, and Rosenberg, Irwin, with Thompson, Jacqueline. *Biomarkers: The 10 Determinants of Aging You Can Control.* New York: Simon & Schuster, 1991.

Fiatarone, Maria A. et al. "High-Intensity Strength Training in Nonagenarians," *Journal of the American Medical Association* 263:3029–3034, 1990.

Food and Nutrition Board: *Recommended Dietary Allowances* (Tenth Edition), Washington, D.C.: National Academy Press, 1989.

Forbes, Gilbert B. "The Adult Decline in Lean Body Mass," *Human Biology* 48:161–173, 1976.

From the Editors of *Men's Health* Magazine. *How Men Stay Young.* Emmaus, Pennsylvania: Rodale Press, 1991.

From the Editors of Prevention Magazine. *Lifespan-Plus.* Emmaus, Pennsylvania: Rodale Press, 1990.

From the Editors of the University of California, Berkeley, Wellness Letter. *The Wellness Encyclopedia.* Boston: Houghton Mifflin Co., 1991.

Goldberg, Alfred L. et al. "Mechanisms of Work-Induced Hypertrophy of Skeletal Muscle," *Medicine and Science in Sports and Exercise* 7:248–261, 1975.

Goldberg, Linn et al. "Changes in Lipid and Lipoprotein Levels After Weight Training," *Journal of the American Medical Association* 252:504–506, 1984.

Goldfinger, S.E. "Good for What Ails You," *Harvard Health Letter* 16(10):1–2, 1991.

Grunewald, Katharine K., and Bailey, Robert S. "Commercially Marketed Supplements for Bodybuilding Athletes," *Sports Medicine* 15:90–103, 1993.

Gwinup, G. et al. "Thickness of Subcutaneous Fat and Activity of Underlying Muscles," *Annals of Internal Medicine* 74:408-441, 1971.

Herbert, Victor, and Barrett, Stephen. *Vitamins and "Health" Foods.* Philadelphia: George F. Stickley Co., 1981.

Hildreth, Suzanne. "Exercise: You Need to Know the Facts . . . to Sell the Benefits," *Club Business International* 10:27-33:65, December 1989.

Hurley, B.F. et al. "Resistive Training Can Reduce Coronary Risk Factors Without Altering VO$_2$ Max or Percent Body Fat," *Medicine and Science in Sports and Exercise* 20:150–154, 1988.

Hutchins, Ken. *Super Slow: The Ultimate Exercise Protocol* (Second Edition). Casselberry, FL: Super Slow Systems, 1992.

Jones, Arthur. *The Lumbar Spine, the Cervical Spine, and the Knee.* Ocala, FL: MedX Corporation, 1993.

_____. *Nautilus Training Principles: Bulletin No. 1.* DeLand, FL: Nautilus Sports/Medical Industries, 1970.

_____. "The Upper Body Squat," *Iron Man* 29:41, 47, 71, June 1970.

Katch, Frank I. et al. "Effects of Sit-Up Exercise Training on Adipose Cell Size and Adiposity," *Research Quarterly for Exercise and Sport* 55:242–247, 1984.

Kelsey, Jennifer L., and White, Augustus A. "Epidemiology and Impact of Low-Back Pain," *Spine* 5:133–142, 1980.

Kerr, Graham. *Graham Kerr's Creative Choices Cookbook.* New York: G.P. Putnam's Sons, 1993.

Keyes, Ancel A. et al. "Basal Metabolism and Age of Adult Man," *Metabolism* 22:579–587, 1973.

Lamb, Lawrence E. *The Weighting Game.* Secaucus, NJ: Lyle Stuart Inc., 1988.

Lambrinides, Ted. "Internal Training: Improving Your Anaerobic Capacity," *High Intensity Training Newsletter* 2:10–12, December 1990.

Mackay, Harvey B. *Sharkproof.* New York: Harper Business, 1993.

Masters, William H. and Johnson, Virginia E. *Human Sexual Response*. Boston: Little, Brown and Company, 1966.

Messier, Stephen P., and Dill, Mary E. "Alterations in Strength and Maximal Oxygen Uptake Consequent to Nautilus Circuit Weight Training," *Research Quarterly for Exercise and Sport* 56:345–351, 1985.

Moscovitz, Judy. *The Dieter's Companion*. New York: Avon Books, 1989.

Pesmen, Curtis. *How a Man Ages*. New York: Ballantine Books, 1984.

Peterson, James A. "Total Conditioning: A Case Study," *Athletic Journal* 56:40–55, September 1975.

Pollock, Michael L. et al. "Muscle," in *Rehabilitation of the Spine* edited by Hochschuler, Richard D. and coeditors. St. Louis: Mosby-Year Book, Inc., 1993.

Robertson, Laurel et al. *The New Laurel's Kitchen*. Berkeley, CA: Ten Speed Press, 1986.

Sizer, Frances, and Whitney, Eleanor. *Nutrition Concepts and Controversies* (Sixth Edition). St. Paul, MN: West Publishing Co., 1994.

Stare, Fredrick A., and Aronson, Virginia. *Food for Fitness After Fifty*. Philadelphia: George F. Stickley Co., 1985.

The Good Health Fact Book. Pleasantville, NY: Reader's Digest Association, 1992.

Todd, Jan. "George Barker Windship and the First Weight-Training Boom," *Iron Game History* 3:3–14, September 1993.

Toufexis, Anastasia. "Drowsy American," *Time* 139:78–83, December 17, 1990.

"Toxic Plants Sold in Health Food Stores," *The Medical Letter*, April 6, 1979.

Tyler, Varro E. *The New Honest Herbal*. Philadelphia: George F. Stickley Co., 1987.

Webb, Wilse B. *Sleep: The Gentle Tyrant* (Second Edition). Boston: Amber Publishing Company, Inc., 1992.

Westcott, Wayne. *Strength Fitness* (Fourth Edition). Dubuque, IA: Wm. C. Brown Publishers, 1995.

Whelan, Elizabeth M., and Stare, Fredrick J. *Panic in the Pantry*. Buffalo, NY: Prometheus Books, 1992.

Zorbas, William S., and Karpovich, Peter V. "The Effect of Weight Lifting Upon the Speed of Muscular Contraction," *Research Quarterly* 22:145–148, 1951.

ABOUT THE AUTHOR

Ellington Darden received his bachelor's and master's degrees in physical education from Baylor University, a doctorate in exercise science from Florida State University, and completed two years of post-doctoral work in food and nutrition.

For 20 years, Dr. Darden was Director of Research of Nautilus Sports/Medical Industries. He has written more than 300 articles for consumer magazines and scientific journals and 42 books on fitness, including *The Nautilus Diet, The Nautilus Book, High-Intensity Home Training, 32 Days to a 32-Inch Waist,* and *The Six-Week Fat-to-Muscle Makeover.*

Dr. Darden travels extensively giving training sessions and workshops to fitness instructors throughout the United States and Canada. He is currently doing research at the Gainesville Health & Fitness Center in Gainesville, Florida.

Just Because You've Finished The Book Doesn't Mean You're Finished.

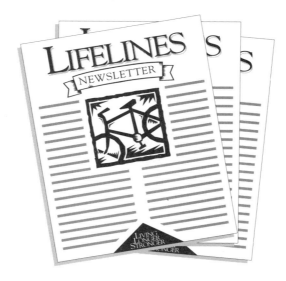

INTRODUCING LIFELINES NEWSLETTER
A Major Breakthrough From Living Longer Stronger.

Keep updated on the most important discoveries and findings in the world of physical fitness, proactive learning, and personal productivity. With Living-Longer-Stronger's *LIFELINES* newsletter, you'll have timely information on how to maintain the momentum you've built from this book for the rest of your life.

Some of the reports will cover the topics of strength training, cardiovascular endurance, fat loss, food and nutrition, sports medicine, and age blocking. You'll find enlightening facts on optimizing the new you. These sections will discuss everything from dressing for success to specially designed Living-Longer-Stronger travel adventures.

LIFELINES will become a permanent part of your personal development library. You'll also get ongoing accounts of Dr. Ellington Darden's cutting-edge research, as he supervises the eating and exercising of numerous experimental groups.

For information on *LIFELINES* subscriptions, please call Lena Lenford at:

1-800-LLS-4YOU
1-800-557-4968

Ellington Darden is available for seminars and telephone consultations.